Biological Aspects of Mental Health Nursing

To my parents who taught me so much – SR

To Alison and Ruth for your love, understanding and keeping me 'mentally healthy' – PM

For Churchill Livingstone:

Senior Commissioning Editor: Jacqueline Curthoys
Project Manager: Gail Murray
Project Development Manager: Dinah Thom
Designer: George Ajayi

Biological Aspects of Mental Health Nursing

A. Shupikai Rinomhota MSc BSc(Hons) RGN RMN PGCE
Cert in Counselling
Nursing Lecturer, School of Healthcare Studies, University of Leeds, Leeds, UK

Paul Marshall PhD BSc RGN RMN CertEd
Senior Nursing Lecturer (Subject Co-ordinator Biological Sciences), School of Healthcare Studies, University of Leeds, Leeds, UK

Foreword by

Kevin Gournay CBE MPhil PhD CPsychol AFBPsS
FRCN RN ENB 650
Professor of Psychiatric Nursing, Institute of Psychiatry, London, UK

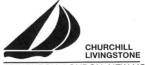

CHURCHILL
LIVINGSTONE
EDINBURGH LONDON NEW YORK PHILADELPHIA ST LOUIS SYDNEY TORONTO 2000

CHURCHILL LIVINGSTONE
An imprint of Harcourt Publishers Limited

© Harcourt Publishers Limited 2000

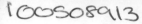 is a registered trademark of Harcourt Publishers Limited

First published 2000

ISBN 0 443 05990 X

British Library Cataloguing in Publication Data
A catalogue record for this book is available from the British Library

Library of Congress Cataloging in Publication Data
A catalog record for this book is available from the Library of
Congress

Note
Medical knowledge is constantly changing. As new information
becomes available, changes in treatment, procedures, equipment and
the use of drugs become necessary. The authors and the publishers
have taken care to ensure that the information given in this text is
accurate and up to date. However, readers are strongly advised to
confirm that the information, especially with regard to drug usage,
complies with the latest legislation and standards of practice.

The
publisher's
policy is to use
paper manufactured
from sustainable forests

Printed in China

Contents

Foreword

There are 57000 mental health nurses on the register of the UKCC who practise in psychiatric settings. In addition to this 57000 there are another 30000 nurses on the UKCC register who practise in other areas. The education and training of this workforce has changed tremendously in the last forty years, and, in that time, the role has changed from that of the attendant, in the custodial setting of the Victorian asylum, to that of the well-trained nurse within a range of settings. At the same time, we now have much greater understanding of the causation of mental illness and we now have a wide range of psychological, social and biological treatments. Today's mental health nurse, therefore, needs a sound knowledge of many and diverse areas. Unfortunately, there are problems with mental health nursing education, and it is my view that there has been a disproportionate amount of emphasis placed on redundant social and psychological theories which have become the hobby horses of some nursing academics. In turn, many university nursing departments are dominated by nursing models which, it has to be said, are based on discredited and out-of-date psychoanalytic theories. Mental health nurses today need up-to-date knowledge of psychological treatments, based on sound experimental evidence, and they also need to know about the biological basis for mental illnesses and understand the underlying science behind pharmacological and other physical treatments. Although it should seem obvious, today's mental health nurse needs to have a knowledge of psychological, social and biological factors involved in the genesis and maintenance of mental illness, and to be able to integrate knowledge from each of these areas so as to understand the nature of the illness and the person in a holistic fashion. This book provides an excellent overview of the neurobiological basis of mental health nursing. While the authors provide no apology for focusing on the biological, they have succeeded in providing an account which integrates this domain with other areas. Indeed, they argue very effectively that an understanding of neurobiological factors is essential to understanding how the equilibrium of mental health is maintained and how, in turn, abnormalities in neurobiology upset the internal balance or homeostasis.

This book is also timely because there are, in my view, key areas where mental health nurses will need to have an increasing focus in years to come. First, it is clear that the biological research into not only major mental illnesses, such as schizophrenia and bipolar affective disorder, but also into panic disorder and obsessive compulsive disorder (OCD), is developing exponentially. Thus, tomorrow's nurses will need to understand this new knowledge, particularly in the area of genetics and neurochemistry. Second, the last two or three years have seen the introduction of a new wave of antipsychotic medication and it is clear there are further new treatments in the pipeline. Nurses need to understand how these medications work and, indeed, to have a comprehensive understanding of possible side effects. Finally, it is clear that prescribing for mental health nurses is a not too distant prospect. There is already dramatic development in this regard in the USA, where every state now has legislation giving nurses prescriptive authority. In mental health nursing, some states allow nurses to prescribe medication independently, although in most states nurses prescribe a full range of medications, either under the supervision of the psychiatrist or in collaboration with a psychiatrist or family physician. Obviously, having such a responsibility provides an imperative for nurses to become much more cognizant of neurobiological principles.

The young, and not so young, people entering mental health nursing today will receive an all round education, and will enter their vocation as professionals, a different profile indeed to that of the attendant of the post-World War Two era. This book should be an essential text for this generation, but hopefully nurses who are already established in their profession could use the pages of this book as a resource to update their skills and knowledge. Finally, this book should help practitioners to provide the patients they care for with a total and holistic approach.

Kevin Gournay CBE

Preface

Mental health nurses have to draw on a broad expanse of knowledge, involving various, and at times seemingly conflicting, disciplines. Mental health nursing has also suffered the fate of the swinging pendulum: over the past two decades the pendulum has swung away from the medical model towards psychosocial and humanistic models with an apparent rejection of anything biological. Thankfully, however, in recent years the pendulum seems to be settling more centrally with the development of biopsychosocial-spiritual models. We make no apologies for taking a biological perspective. We believe that, alongside other disciplines and perspectives, mental health nurses should seriously consider the biological aspects of mental health problems and the associated implications for the client, families and the nurse. We have tried to provide a broad overview of the biological factors that may contribute to, and may arise from, the development of mental health problems. We have also tried to identify issues that are clearly relevant for mental health nurses. Naturally, we have had to be selective, and it may be that we have missed out, with hindsight, some very obvious topics. For this we can only apologise.

Over the past two decades there has been a remarkable explosion in the understanding of the biological basis of the brain and behaviour; in particular in the technology used for imaging and studying whole brain as well as neuronal activity. Furthermore, developments in pharmacological therapeutic approaches continue at a tremendous rate. For reasons of selectivity and to keep an appropriate focus, we have been able only to touch on some of these areas. Finally, we have only referred briefly to specific nursing interventions and strategies as appropriate. Again, this may be a disappointment for some but this has been deliberate. There are many excellent nursing texts available but very few address in-depth biological aspects. We can only hope that we have presented issues that we regard as important for mental health nurses in a way that is readable and interesting for the reader. We hope that this book may stimulate colleagues to read more extensively and to consider the basis for the nursing strategies adopted.

Shupi Rinomhota
Paul Marshall

Leeds 2000

Acknowledgements

We would like to acknowledge the generous assistance of Dr C. Taylor, Dr M. Glass, Dr L. Pieri and Ms L. Mathews in the development of the case studies, and Dr C. Ramchard for his challenging and helpful comments along the way.

The quest for holistic care in theory and practice

The need for a comprehensive basis of nursing assessment (diagnosis), planning, implementation and evaluation of nursing actions requires a good understanding of the knowledge associated with body responses to illness. Whichever philosophy and model of nursing care delivery practitioners choose to adopt and use, both practitioners and clients or patients need to understand how to manage discomfort. This understanding is enhanced further by our knowledge of the body's potential and actual responses to illness. Does a knowledge of biological sciences help practitioners in mental health nursing without becoming too medically orientated? If one answers this question positively, then the next question that one is bound to ask is: what exactly do mental health nurses need to know and which aspects of biological sciences knowledge are relevant to mental health nursing?

THE ONGOING DEBATE

McCrone (1996) argues that one of the greatest challenges facing mental health nurses today is to recognise the knowledge developed through the evolution of biological psychiatry and to integrate such knowledge into their own practice. The human body existed long before the discipline of medicine was developed. Implicit in the previous statement is the fact that the quest to have any knowledge about the human body is not part of the process of medicalisation but a genuine professional attempt to understand how pathological changes and environmental influences affect the body's homeostatic mechanisms and alter thought processes, emotions and behaviour.

Barker (1999) states that he 'harbours a great dread that the ambition to explain all of human life through complex biological and neurochemical models will turn the world of psychiatry into a truly mindless enterprise' (p 24). However, he accepts that 'the brain, despite its amazing complexity, devotes most of its life to processing and reorganising information from the world beyond our skulls – the world experience' (Barker 1999, p 24). Munro (1999) supports Barker's view by saying that 'biological determinism has run riot in psychiatry' and goes on to say that there is no longer the desire to understand whole persons in their social contexts but rather a desire to 'realign our patient's neurotransmitters'.

It does appear that there are several anomalies in the arguments that are put forward against a knowledge of biological sciences by mental health nurses. The first anomaly is that whole persons can only be understood in a social context. What exactly is a whole person, we would like to ask? There is no doubt that to understand an individual person, one needs to know the social and cultural influences under which that individual functions, but this does not invalidate the fact that there can be pathophysiological changes and external environmental factors that can affect the totality of individual functioning.

The second anomaly that seems to exist is that of the notion of the mind. What is the mind and how does the mind operate? Many advocates against the acquisition of biological knowledge by mental health nurses seem to have failed to understand a very important aspect of the mind–brain interface. Wherever there is an input there is an output. The role of the brain to receive, interpret, process, integrate, coordinate and store information is well accepted, even by those who are anti-biology. What is not appreciated and understood by many people is how the mind–brain interface affects the totality of output that we all interpret as personality, thoughts, feelings, behaviour and many other attributes that make each individual unique. Indeed if without the brain there is no individual, as Barker (1999) accepts, then it stands to reason to accept that the brain has an important role in shaping the chapters and life script of each individual, at least in this existence.

The third anomaly that is rampant is that a knowledge of biological sciences by mental health nurses will make them cease to care for mentally ill people adequately. This anomaly is fuelled by the added belief that the cure–care models are incompatible. Baumann et al (1998) argue that cure and care are not mutually exclusive but that they are endpoints on a continuum that is used by all health care workers and that, under different clinical situations, different combinations of cure and care are appropriate. Knowledge of biological sciences by mental health nurses does not interfere with their ability to care. If anything, such knowledge should make mental health nurses more competent carers and more holistic in their approach since they will be working from a knowledge base. Munro (1999) suggests that biological knowledge allows mental health nurses to condone and promote the widespread overuse and misuse of toxic chemicals which have long-term side effects such as tardive dyskinesia.

Nurses who believe only in the psychosocial and psychodynamic models of care to the total exclusion of others and who are strongly opposed to knowledge of biological sciences are unlikely to have the necessary knowledge to support those mentally ill individuals who do need their medication in addition to other supportive intervention techniques. Nurses need to be able to distinguish the presenting features of an illness from the side effects of drugs. This is particularly important where nurses are working alone in the community and may be the only health care professional that a mentally ill person sees regularly. This view of nurses frequently claiming that their practice is holistic even though they devalue the acquisition and use of biological sciences knowledge has been challenged by other authors (Clarke 1995, Trnobranski 1993) who see the acquisition of biological knowledge as a basis for safe practice. We take the same view that there is no holistic nursing where the practitioner is not knowledgeable or is dismissive about biological issues. This does not mean that such practice is invalid, but it is certainly not holistic. Indeed we propose that where nursing care is inadequate this may very well have to do with limited holistic knowledge by mental health nurses as well as inadequacies in resources.

The fourth anomaly that seems to exist is that put forward by Clarke (1999), who suggests that there are no biological issues in human experience. A food intolerance or an allergy from an unknown food substance by an individual is a human experience. Likewise hallucinations, low mood, side-effects from therapeutic drugs, confusion, constipation and restlessness to mention but a few are all human experiences that have a biological perspective. To understand human experiences adequately, not only do nurses need to listen actively to the stories being told by each individual but they also need to have both broad-based and specific knowledge on many different issues that add an understanding to the whole school of life.

RATIONALE FOR HOLISTIC CARE

This book is not about the molecules that 'make people mad', but about concepts that we believe individual nurses will find relevant to their practice, whichever sphere of mental health nursing they are engaged in. We do not believe that psychobiological models are necessarily reductionist in approach since it is how the various issues discussed are related to the whole functioning of the individual whatever the individual circumstances that constitutes holistic practice. The views and arguments on the genetic basis of some mental illnesses (Gournay 1995, 1996, 1998) are quite valid though they have come under criticism from others (Dawson 1994, 1997) because the issues that need to be clarified are what predisposes individuals to mental illness and how best to intervene and support such individuals. The fact that there is no viable model for normal and abnormal thought processes, as Dawson (1997) points out, does not mean that we should stop research into our understanding of the possible causes of mental illness, whatever they may be, including biological ones.

New approaches to care delivery such as interpersonal psychotherapy (Martin, 1999), which encompasses both a biological and psychological approach to nursing practice, are what mental health nurses should be considering and adopting instead of remaining in the citadels of age-old beliefs and ideals. The arguments by Martin (1999) on the effective use of interpersonal psychotherapy are supported by earlier studies by Elkin et al (1989), in which interpersonal psychotherapy was found to be therapeutically more effective than cognitive behavioural therapy. Modern imaging techniques such as single photon emission computed tomography (SPECT) and positron emission tomography (PET) have helped to clarify some of the pathophysiological issues in vivo in humans. However, for caring to be good, it must be directed at the right things and in the right way (Allmark 1998) but such caring will not be achieved until all aspects of the individual are considered. Babich (1992) argues that an emphasis on biological psychiatric nursing will continue to be needed until psychiatric mental health nurses have as good an understanding of the physiodynamics as they do the psychodynamics of mental illness. Earlier, Guze (1989) stated that the role of a biopsychosocial model was to view biological and genetic sciences in interplay with the environment, learning and culture in the growth and development of all forms of life, including human beings.

Peplau (1994) quite rightly points out that innovations in practice arise from the findings of nursing research, from changes within health care systems and/or from new demands in society. She also reports evidence that psychiatric mental health nurses are spending their time giving medication, recording it in patient charts and observing for compliance and complications at the expense of talking to patients. Again we argue that where this is occurring, there is a return to custodial care and nurses have failed to understand their roles, and there is also a case for resources being inadequate. It is interesting to note that Peplau (1994) acknowledges that genetic predisposition, biochemical imbalances and pathophysiological factors play a significant part in mental illness and that it would be foolish to dismiss this role, no matter how small. Both liaison psychiatry issues and dual diagnosis (Smith & Hucker 1994) where substance abuse is implicated are already posing new challenges to mental health nurses.

We agree with Peplau (1994) that the nature–nurture debate has a long history and that it will never go away. If indeed there is a swing to nature, as many authors have pointed out, we argue that the real challenge for mental health nurses in the 21st century is to blend the nature–nurture routes as part of a strategy to understand the mind–brain interface and to understand individuals from a holistic perspective.

THE CHALLENGE

It is a fair assumption to say that most educationists subscribe fully to the notion that as new knowledge comes to light, there is a need to set an arena for the understanding and application of this newly acquired knowledge, followed by its analysis, synthesis and evaluation. The application of newly acquired biological knowledge can only be achieved when both practitioners and students are able, as Clarke (1995) points out, to articulate the relevance of biological science as an important basis for nursing care if true holistic care is to be achieved. We subscribe to Cannon's (1929) view, and it is our own belief as well, that the study of particular activities of the various parts of the body has progressed and will continue to do so to a greater extent than is recognised by many people. This study will facilitate an in-depth understanding of the interplay between the various parts that constitute the organism as well as the interplay between the organism and its environment. The challenge that is here now for mental health nurses and other professionals is to bring the quest for delivering holistic care in practice to its logical conclusion through an understanding of all the facets that make each individual unique.

It is our hope that the various neuroanatomy, neuroimaging, neurochemistry, hormonal, genetic, nutritional, immunological and psychopharmacological issues that are discussed in the chapters of this book will enrich the mental health nurse to be the patient's advocate from a base that is rooted in knowledge, understanding and application. This is much more effective than adopting an anti-biology and anti-psychiatry stance that is based on emotional hype, personal orientation and bias.

REFERENCES

Allmark P 1998 Is caring a virtue? Journal of Advanced Nursing 28(3): 466–472
Babich K 1992 What is biological psychiatry? How will the trend toward biological psychiatry affect the future role of the psychiatric mental health nurse? Journal of Psychosocial Nursing 30(1): 33–35
Barker P 1999 Growing from experience. Nursing Times 95(33): 24
Baumann A O, Deber R B, Silverman B E, Mallette C M 1998 Who cares? Who cures? The ongoing debate in the provision of healthcare. Journal of Advanced Nursing 28(5): 1040–1045
Cannon W B 1929 Organization for physiological homeostasis. Physiological Reviews IX(3): 399–431
Clarke L 1999 Nursing in search of a science: the rise and rise of the new nurse brutalism. Mental Health Care 21(8): 270–272
Clarke M 1995 Nursing and the biological sciences. Journal of Advanced Nursing 22: 405–406
Dawson P J 1994 Contra biology: a polemic. Journal of Advanced Nursing 20: 1094–1103
Dawson P J 1997 A reply to Kevin Gournay's 'Schizophrenia: a review of the contemporary literature and implications for mental health nursing theory, practice and education'. Journal of Psychiatric and Mental Health Nursing 4: 1–7
Elkin I, Shea M T, Watkins J T et al 1989 National Institute of Mental Health treatment of depression collaborative research programme: general effectiveness of treatments. Archives of General Psychiatry 46(11): 971–982
Gournay K 1995 New facts on schizophrenia. Nursing Times 91(25): 32–33

Gournay K 1996 Schizophrenia: a review of the contemporary literature and implications for mental health nursing theory, practice and education. Journal of Psychiatric and Mental Health Nursing 3: 7–12

Gournay K 1998 Face to face. Nursing Times 94: 40–41

Guze S B 1989 Biological psychiatry: is there any other kind? Psychological Medicine 19: 315–323

McCrone S H 1996 The impact of the evolution of biological psychiatry on psychiatric nursing. Journal of Psychosocial Nursing 34(1): 38–46

Martin E 1999 Switched on. Nursing Times 95(36): 52–53

Munro R 1999 There is sin in them there genes. Nursing Times 95(33): 28–29

Peplau H E 1994 Psychiatric mental health nursing: challenge and change. Journal of Psychiatric and Mental Health Nursing 1: 3–7

Smith J, Hucker S 1994 Schizophrenia and substance abuse. British Journal of Psychiatry 165: 13–21

Trnobranski P H 1993 Biological sciences and the curriculum: a challenge for educationalists. Journal of Advanced Nursing 18: 493–499

2

The concept of homeostasis

The constancy or stability of the internal environment is the condition for free life.

(Claude Bernard, 1857)

Key Points

- Homeostasis is the maintenance of a stable internal environment
- The internal environment refers to extracellular fluid
- Internal and external challenges cause deviation from the norm and trigger self-regulating processes
- Feedback mechanisms continually report the status of the internal environment to the control centre
- Holistic nursing is about facilitating the restoration of internal well-being in clients who we work with
- Internal well-being means a stable internal environment
- Holistic nursing care aims to restore physical, emotional and spiritual homeostasis
- Identification and reduction of risk factors promote homeostasis

Currently, homeostasis is a term that is used to represent a view of biological health and is therefore an important concept in both biology and nursing (Rinomhota & Cooper 1996). An individual's state of physical fitness and mental well-being are good indicators of effective homeostatic function. According to Chiras (1995) there is a very close link between human health and the environment and from this can be drawn the conclusion that the body's homeostastic function serves as an indicator of the quality of the environment in which individuals live. This chapter explores the concept of homeostasis and aspects of physical and mental well-being with particular emphasis on the role and quality of the environment in influencing homeostatic function.

FOUNDERS OF THE HOMEOSTATIC CONCEPT

The term *homeostasis* is derived from two Greek words, *homeo* meaning staying the same and *stasis* meaning standing still (Tortora & Grabowski 1993). Our current knowledge of homeostasis has its foundation in the work of Claude Bernard (1813–1878), a French scientist, and Walter

7

Bradford Cannon (1871–1945), an American neurologist and physiologist. Their work was significant in helping to clarify the issues surrounding homeostasis.

Claude Bernard was born in 1813 in Saint-Julien and died in 1878 in Paris. After medical school, Bernard worked as a research assistant under François Magendie, on spinal nerves, the role of gastric juice in nutrition, neurology and metabolism (Encyclopaedia Britannica 1988a). Bernard helped to establish the principles of experimentation in life sciences and is now regarded as one of the founders of experimental medicine. Bernard discovered the role of the pancreas in digestion and found that the secretions of the pancreas digest lipid molecules into fatty acids and glycerol. His work on the pancreas led him to discover the role of the liver in storing glucose as glycogen. Bernard's greatest contribution was his idea of the internal environment of the organism which has led to our present understanding of the concept of homeostasis. In 1857 he wrote: 'La fixité du milieu enterieur est la condition de la vie libre' whose translation is 'the constancy of the internal environment is the condition for free life' (Roberts 1986).

Walter Bradford Cannon was born in 1871 in Prairie du Chien, Wisconsin, and died in 1945 in Franklin, New Hampshire. He was the first person to use X-rays in physiological studies and investigated haemorrhagic and traumatic shock reactions during the First World War. Cannon studied the autonomic nervous system and discovered sympathin, an adrenaline-like substance liberated at the end of certain nerve cells, and he also worked on methods of blood storage (Encyclopaedia Britannica 1988b). In 1915 he published his work on *Bodily Changes in Pain, Hunger, Fear and Rage* which was followed by *The Wisdom of the Body* in 1932. Cannon was the first person to use the term *homeostasis*.

WHAT IS HOMEOSTASIS?

Homeostasis is the maintenance of a stable internal environment. It is a self-regulating process by which biological systems tend to maintain stability while adjusting to conditions that are optimal for survival and responding to stressors that challenge that stability. Successful regulation of homeostasis allows life to continue, whereas disruption of homeostatic regulation leads to illness, dysfunction, disease or death.

THE INTERNAL ENVIRONMENT

In order to appreciate homeostatic mechanisms, an understanding of the concept of the internal environment is essential. The internal environment refers to the composition of the extracellular fluid, which is made up of two components: interstitial fluid (intercellular fluid) and plasma (or blood). But in addition to these, there are also other fluid environments such as cerebrospinal fluid (CSF), transcellular fluid and synovial fluid.

> Internal environment = Extracellular fluid = Intercellular fluid + Plasma (blood)

Many components of the internal environment do not keep to a fixed value but adapt to changing requirements. These characteristics, therefore, are regulated rather than controlled since control implies maintenance of a fixed value. The characteristics regulated include body temperature, water, pH levels, nutrients such as glucose, amino acids, vitamins, fatty acids and glycerol, oxygen, electrolytes and waste products such as carbon dioxide, urea and creatinine. Urea is a product of protein metabolism that occurs mostly in the liver while creatinine results from muscle mass or muscle protein metabolism. Very simply, in order to permit bursts of activity, a large amount of phosphate is stored as phosphocreatine. Phosphocreatine has approximately the same amount of free energy of hydrolysis (i.e. when broken down) as adenosine triphosphate (ATP). During bursts of activity, phosphocreatine is broken down to release its energy resulting in the formation of creatinine. Importantly, the three fluid compartments interact and affect each other. The concentration of substances in the intercellular fluid directly affects the concentration of substances in the cells, while the concentration of substances in blood directly affects the concentration of substances in intercellular fluid (Tudor & Tudor 1985).

A classic example of this is the exchange of water between plasma, intercellular fluid and the intracellular environment. Excessive ingestion of water, as can sometimes occur with disorders of thought and perception, can lead to fluid leaving the plasma and entering the intercellular space. This can result in a fall in the osmolality of the intercellular fluid relative to inside the cells. This in turn would result in the movement of water from the intercellular space into the cells due to the effects of osmosis, resulting in cell oedema and cell dysfunction. The brain cells in particular are vulnerable to changes in cell water content, and cerebral oedema can lead to dizziness, mental confusion, seizures, unconsciousness and, in the worst case scenario, to death. Failure to regulate or maintain a stable internal environment results in the accumulation of toxins, alteration of cell pH, alteration of cell fluid content, disruption of cellular and tissue activity and cell death, and is a threat to life.

OPEN AND CLOSED SYSTEMS

Some non-biological systems are closed, which makes them static. An example of this is a solution in a sealed test tube. Other systems are open and this makes them dynamic. Biological systems are of the open type. When a system in dynamic equilibrium is disturbed, inbuilt regulatory devices respond to the departures (feedback) to establish a new balance and the system tends eventually to reach a steady state. A steady state is a balance that resists change from outside forces. Thus, homeostasis is not a static balance but a dynamic equilibrium in which continuous change occurs and yet relatively uniform conditions prevail.

STRUCTURAL AND FUNCTIONAL REQUIREMENTS FOR HOMEOSTASIS

Any operational system requires several structural features to be in place for efficient function. Likewise, for homeostasis to occur, several structural features need to be in place.

Receptors

There is a need to detect the stimulus, which is achieved by the presence of receptors. There are many different types of receptors which can be classified by location or by stimulus detected (Table 2.1).

Table 2.1 Receptors

Location	Specific receptors	Responsive to:
Exteroreceptors	Nociceptors	Noxious chemical and mechanical stimulus
	Thermoreceptors	Heat
	Photoreceptors	Light
	Chemoreceptors	Smell
	Mechanoreceptors	Pressure
Enteroreceptors (visceroreceptors)	Baroreceptors	Pressure (e.g. arterial blood pressure)
	Chemoreceptors	Oxygen and carbon dioxide partial pressures
	Nociceptors	Noxious chemical and mechanical stimulus
	Osmoreceptors	Plasma solute concentration (osmolarity)
Proprioceptors	Muscle spindle (mechanorecepetors)	Stretching of muscle
	Golgi tendon organ (mechanoreceptor)	Stretching of tendons
	Mechanoreceptors	Joint movement

Classification by location

When using location for classification, receptors can be *exteroceptors, enteroceptors (visceroceptors)* or *proprioceptors*. Exteroceptors are located at or near the surface of the body and provide information about the external environment since they are sensitive to stimuli outside the body. They transmit messages of hearing, sight, smell, touch, pressure, temperature and pain. Enteroceptors (visceroceptors) are located in blood vessels and internal organs (the viscera) and provide information about the internal environment. Sensations arise from within the body and may be felt as pain, pressure, hunger, thirst, fatigue and nausea. Proprioceptors are located in muscles, tendons, joints and the inner ear and provide information about body position and movement. Sensations give information about muscle tension, the position and activity of joints and equilibrium.

Classification by stimulus detected

Mechanoreceptors detect deformation of the receptor itself or in adjacent cells. Stimuli detected include touch, pressure, vibration, proprioception, hearing, equilibrium and blood pressure. *Thermoreceptors* detect temperature changes while *photoreceptors* detect light on the retina of the eye. The detection of taste in the mouth, smell in the nose and chemicals in body fluids such as oxygen, carbon dioxide and glucose is achieved by *chemoreceptors*. *Nociceptors* detect pain usually as a result of physical or/and chemical damage to tissues. *Osmoreceptors* are sensitive to water changes in the body.

One aspect that may need to be considered by mental health workers is the possible role of altered receptor function and how this may be related to hallucinations. Studies by Hoffman (1999) used a technique called masked speech tracking in which subjects are required to track narrative speech whose phonetic clarity is reduced by use of superimposed multispeaker babble. Hoffman's studies showed that neuroanatomical pathology in which networks are altered by reducing connections within the working memory module or arrangement coupled by a hyperdopaminergic state leads to a situation in which spontaneous word percepts are produced in the absence of any phonetic input. This is supported by Dolan et al (1999) who, using functional neuroimaging techniques such as positron emmission tomography (PET), highlighted a disturbance in neural interactions in schizophrenia. Further evidence is provided in a review by David (1999) in which he describes the disinhibition model, whereby reduced sensory input results in cortical activity being experienced as hallucinations, and a cerebral irritation model that suggests abnormal cortical excitability in areas associated with sensory memory.

In the review by David (1999), the experience of auditory verbal hallucinations has been associated with neural activity by using PET, single photon emission computed tomography (SPECT) and functional magnetic resonance imaging (MRI) together with work on in vivo receptor binding for dopamine and gamma-amino butyric acid (GABA).

There is evidence to suggest that disordered function of receptors results in failure of the appropriate response being produced, as seen in several pathological conditions such as pseudohypoparathyroidism and nephrogenic diabetes insipidus whereby parathyroid hormone and vaso-pressin fail to stimulate an increased production in cyclic adenosine monophosphate (AMP) in their target cells, which they do in normal individuals (Ganong 1989). Antibodies against thyroid stimulating hormone receptors result in Graves' disease (exophthalmic goitre) characterised by an enlarged goitre and protrusion of eyeballs, while antibodies against nicotinic acetylcholine receptors cause myasthenia gravis.

Information carriers

Once detected, the message is transmitted via nerves or blood to and/or from a control centre which may be the spinal cord or the brain.

Information processor (control centre)

The part of the central nervous system (CNS) that receives and integrates all information arriving from other parts of the CNS is called the control centre. The control centre can be part of the brain or spinal cord and within it are physiological limits or ranges known as set points.

Effectors

Following processing of information by the control centre, an output is sent to effectors. Effectors can be muscles, organs or glands. They receive information from the control centre and produce a response to the stimulus. It is the effector's response that will attempt to correct the deviation from the set point.

Thus the requirements for a basic homeostatic mechanism will include the stimulus, a receptor, a transmission mechanism, a control centre, an effector, a response and a feedback mechanism as illustrated in Figure 2.1.

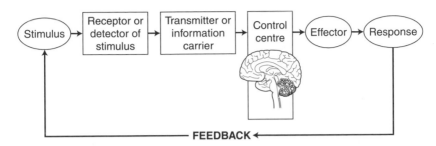

Figure 2.1   Requirements for homeostasis.

FEEDBACK MECHANISMS

Any challenge to a biological process will cause inbuilt regulatory devices to respond to departures from the set point so that a new balance can be established. Feedback mechanisms refer to the continual reporting of situations to the control area. A feedback mechanism can be either negative or positive.

In negative feedback the output counteracts the input. This means that the output reverses the direction of the initial condition. The situation in negative feedback is *stimulatory-inhibitory*. Negative feedback results in

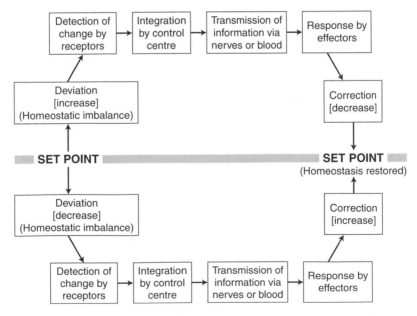

Figure 2.2   Negative feedback shown by correction of deviation. Reproduced from Rinomhota & Cooper (1996) with permission of the British Journal of Nursing.

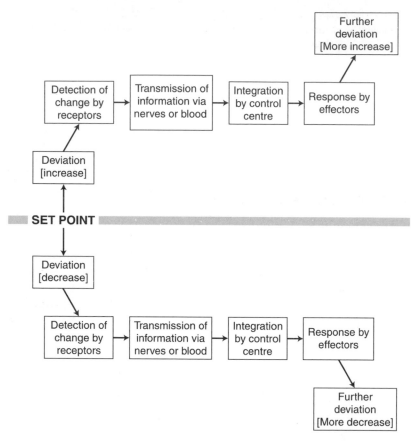

Figure 2.3 Positive feedback shown by further deviation. Adapted from Rinomhota & Cooper (1996) with permission of the British Journal of Nursing.

stability of the internal environment and the maintenance of good health (Fig. 2.2). Positive feedback, on the other hand, results in the output intensifying the input. This means that the output increases the direction of the initial condition further. This situation is *stimulatory-stimulatory*. Positive feedback results in discomfort, ill health, disease or death (Fig. 2.3). Thus, with a few exceptions such as the increased release of oxytocin during parturition until birth is achieved and the cascade system of clotting factors until blood clotting occurs, positive feedback is not desirable physiologically.

THE PHENOMENON OF INBUILT ERROR

The homeostatic response to internal and external challenges is never 100% efficient. Implicit in this statement is that some degree of error is

fundamental to control systems (Rinomhota & Cooper 1996). It is important to remember that this degree of error increases as individuals get
older (Clancy & McVicar 1995), when individuals are ill or when the
challenge exceeds the capacity to cope (Rinomhota & Cooper 1996).

REGULATION AND MAINTENANCE OF HOMEOSTASIS

The nervous and endocrine systems are responsible for biological communication and therefore are of prime importance in the regulation of
homeostasis. The nervous system is responsible for short-term regulation
of homeostasis while the endocrine system plays a role in long-term regulation. The nervous system is discussed in detail in Chapter 3 while
some aspects of endocrine function in relation to mental health nursing
are explored in later chapters. In this chapter the role of the brainstem,
hypothalamus, cortex and limbic system are introduced in relation to
their physiological and emotional homeostatic function (Fig. 2.4). A more
in-depth discussion of the function of these structures is presented in
Chapter 3.

It is generally agreed by both biologists and psychologists that in
humans and other mammals, a group of nuclei found deep in the brain

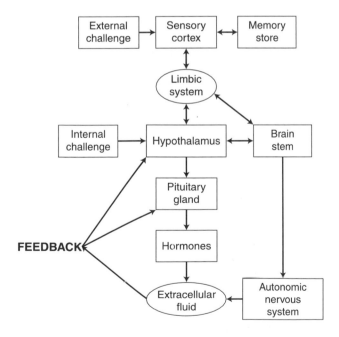

Figure 2.4 The physiological and emotional regulatory mechanisms in homeostasis.
Reproduced from Rinomhota & Cooper (1996) with permission of the British Journal of
Nursing.

form what is known as the limbic system. This system is closely interconnected with the hypothalamus and the brainstem in function. The limbic system modifies the actions of the hypothalamus and the brainstem and is also involved in the expression of emotional behaviour (Atkinson et al 1993), which includes rage, anger, aggression, hostility, fear, sorrow and pleasure. Hole (1993) states that the limbic system is sensitive to upsets in a person's physical or psychological condition that might threaten life.

The endocrine system exerts its effect through the production of hormones which travel to their target or place of action via blood. This means that the endocrine system is often slow in producing its effects. Thus homeostasis is maintained through short-term regulation by the nervous system and through longer-term regulation by the endocrine system. For example, the effects of the nervous system are often seen within milliseconds while those of the endocrine system may take hours, days or weeks. The maintenance of homeostasis, on the other hand, is achieved by the participation, cooperation and interdependency of all the systems of the body. Sherwood (1993) emphasises the interdependent relationship of cells, body systems and homeostasis in that homeostasis is essential for the survival of cells, body systems maintain homeostasis and cells make up body systems. Figure 2.4 illustrates the physiological and emotional homeostatic response mechanisms to both external and internal challenges.

CARTESIAN PHILOSOPHY AND REDUCTIONISM

Prior to the work of Bernard and Cannon, in the 17th century Rene Descartes (1596–1650) contributed to the development of Cartesian philosophy, which brought to the fore the problem of the relationship between mind and body (Russell 1989). Cartesian dualism stated that the mental and physical worlds were separate, and this approach has been fundamental to the development of the biomedical model of health. This dualism was extended by the positivistic philosophers of the 19th century such as Ernst Mach (1838–1916), who advocated the reductionist approach (Russell 1989). The reductionist approach involves the belief that any particular event or phenomenon can be understood as nothing more than the sum of its parts (Atkinson et al 1993, Hayes 1994). This means that in order to understand something, all one has to do is find out its constituent parts and add them all together. One of the main problems with this approach is that the final product is often more than the sum of its parts. 'There is more to understanding the whole than simply analysing its parts, although looking at the parts can often be helpful' (Hayes 1994, p 221).

It is important to mention here that reductionism is associated not only with the biomedical model but also with psychology and sociology, as there are psychological reductionism and social reductionism. Both the biomedical model and the reductionist approach are rejected by most of the nursing profession and all those who believe in a holistic approach to health care (Colaizzi 1975, Pearson & Vaughan 1989, Wilson-Barnett & Batehup 1988). Within the expanded understanding of the concepts of homeostasis presented in this chapter, both the biomedical model and the reductionist approach are rejected.

MENTAL WELL-BEING

Mental homeostasis suggests mental well-being. But what is mental well-being? Any definition of mental health may reflect the perspective of the person defining the term with regard to the aetiology of mental illness. Therefore it can be argued that mental health is just as much a social construct as mental illness.

Mental health refers to the ability of individuals to 'respond adaptively to external and internal stressors' (Antai-Otong 1995, p 120). There is broad agreement that the key components of mental health include:

- the ability to respond effectively to stress
- the capacity to tolerate anxiety, stress and frustration and to delay gratification of needs (impulse control)
- the capacity to appraise events and situations in one's world realistically and objectively (Antai-Otong 1995, p 120).

Menninger (1963) has depicted mental health as successful adaptation that maintains homeostasis or equilibrium and the physiochemical state. Others (Hedlund & Jeffrey 1993, p 2) have given another view in which they state 'evidence of mental health is usually manifested by physical health; meaningful work; enjoyment of life; satisfying relationships with others; and the ability to make sound judgements and decisions; to accept responsibility for one's actions; to give and receive, and to express feelings appropriately'.

Thus from the various perspectives given it could be deduced that mental well-being includes such notions as ability to have rational thought, ability to perceive surroundings and interpret stimuli appropriately, ability to make appropriate choices, sense of hope and purpose, capacity to cope with challenges of daily activity, sense of fulfilment, ability to enter into meaningful relationships and a positive view of self and the future.

HOMEOSTASIS IN HEALTH CARE

Under stress conditions, homeostasis is disturbed and processes are set in motion to correct the disequilibrium (Atkinson et al 1993). These same authors state that the homeostatic framework is very much associated with two aspects of motivation, namely need and drive. They describe a need as any substantial physiological departure from the ideal value and add that the psychological counterpart of a need is a drive which can be described as an aroused state or urge that results from the need. For example, the physiological need that arises when blood glucose levels fall below a set point or ideal value results in this physiological imbalance being corrected by glycogen in liver and muscle being converted to sugar and released into the bloodstream automatically. However, when the physiological mechanisms are unable to maintain a balanced glucose state as determined by the set point, a drive is activated resulting in the aroused organism taking action to restore the balance, such as seeking food.

The need–drive scenario can be thought of with regard to other aspects of the internal environment that need to be regulated such as body temperature, water balance, blood pressure and many others, as already stated in this chapter. Understanding this need–drive relationship is crucial as it helps with an understanding of both the physiological mechanisms and the behavioural adjustments that are adopted by the body and the individual in order to correct any imbalance that may occur physically and/or emotionally.

Egan (1990) describes emotional scenarios in which individuals may find themselves. These emotional scenarios are no different from physiological changes occurring in the body. The *present scenario* equates to the current physical and emotional status of the individual; the *preferred scenario* is akin to the set point or ideal state (i.e. the state at which the body will function at its optimum or the individual at his/her optimum). *Getting there* refers to the corrective mechanisms (physiologically and behaviourally) that are adopted to produce physical and emotional stability.

One common oversight and oversimplification that occurs within the mental health arena is getting hooked on the behavioural aspects only and being oblivious to the complex but fascinating interdependence of the body and the mind. It is important to remember that there is no mind–body dualism. While some of the behaviours exhibited by patients within mental health nursing environments are part of the illness and are rooted in physiological disequilibrium, other behaviours are the result of an attempt to re-establish the internal environmental stability that has been lost.

To put things into perspective, an example of the bipolar condition of manic depression is given here. Manic depression is a bipolar condition characterised by alternate periods of mania and depression as illustrated in Figures 2.5 and 2.6. The preferred scenario is a state of emotional well-being while the present scenario could be a manic or a depressive episode. During both the manic and the depressive phases changes with-

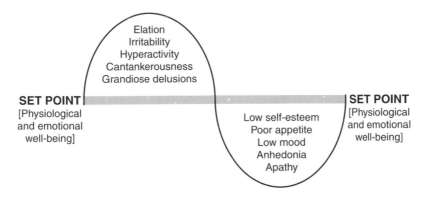

Figure 2.5 The oscillatory nature of a bipolar condition.

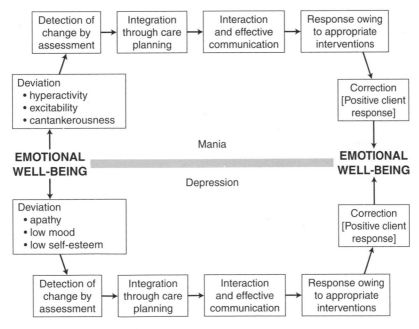

Figure 2.6 Homeostatic regulation in manic depression. Reproduced from Rinomhota & Cooper (1996) with permission of the British Journal of Nursing.

in the internal environment can include electrolyte imbalance, water imbalance, hormonal changes, altered neurotransmitter function and altered nutritional intake.

Clinical nurses spend most of their time communicating with patients, practising comfort measures (doing for) and maximising patients' participation in and control of their own recovery (Benner 1984). Although the actual environment in which nursing care is given and the specific actions of each nurse involved may be different, the roles adopted by different nurses working in different settings have the common objective of facilitating each patient to return to emotional and physical homeostatic balance.

Within a mental health arena some examples of what could be considered as a breakdown in mental homeostasis are: the intense feelings exhibited by an individual suffering from schizophrenia, who may end up showing bizarre behaviour because of what the voices may be saying; the agitation and restlessness shown by an anxious patient; the compulsive thoughts that may result in the continual washing of hands; and the feelings of guilt and hopelessness experienced by a person with depression. The homeostatic mechanisms involved in manic depression are considered in Figure 2.6 and relate to the oscillatory cycle given in Figure 2.5.

Hans Selye's (1974, 1976) fascination with 'the syndrome of just being sick' led him to his research on stress. He reminds the reader that, whatever the illness being experienced by the individual, there are common characteristics of sickness and there are non-specific aspects of stress. The effects of some psychosocial factors, such as divorce and the stress of caring for family members, on the immune system have been studied by Kiecott-Glaser & Glaser (1991) who found that there was diminished immunity. The immune system is known to influence the function of the nervous system via cytokines and other peptides secreted by immune cells (Dunn 1995).

In their discussion on circadian rhythms, Clancy & McVicar (1994) conclude that the psychophysiological well-being of the person results from an integration of physiological function and the consequences of social influences. All these issues support the view that physical and psychosocial challenges, whether they be specific or non-specific, result in alteration of the internal environment and lead to inefficient performance by the individual. Basically, however one chooses to describe or define stress, the actual experience appears to be a common human experience whatever the circumstances. Hoover & Parnell (1984) argue that 'inpatients on a psychiatric-mental health unit have come to a point where their stress is mismanaged to a dysfunctional degree, or they have not developed adequate coping skills for the amount of stress they are experiencing'. This dysfunctional state of affairs may be interpreted by mental health nurses as a breakdown of homeostasis, and the coping strategies that patients develop to manage the challenges are similar to the corrective mechanisms in negative feedback which strive to restore internal environment stability.

Peplau (1952, 1988) discusses the various roles that nurses may adopt in any one working day. It is important to emphasise that the roles adopted by nurses in their day-to-day interactions with patients, whether this be as a stranger, technical expert, counsellor, educator, surrogate, leader or resource person, facilitate the establishment of physical and emotional homeostasis. It is important to state here that the social, intellectual and spiritual aspects of the patient are closely related to this physical and emotional homeostasis.

Nursing is about the promotion of homeostasis. It is concerned with the re-establishment of the stability of the internal environment. It is about promoting those aspects of the caring process as discussed by Swanson (1991) which include caring, knowing, being with, doing for, enabling and maintaining belief. It is about promoting the well-being of patients.

Chiras (1995) put forward a model whereby the concept of homeostasis can be illustrated as a continuum from poorest to best health (Fig. 2.7). An individual in poorest health shows obvious disease or illness while an individual in best health has no disease or illness. From a nursing assessment and a health promotional perspective, individuals showing many risk factors have poor fitness, are in poorest health and will show obvious disease or illness.

The continuum moves from poorest health (many risk factors) via poor health (more risk factors) through good health (a few risk factors) to best health where there are no risk factors, no disease or illness and good fitness. Poorest health represents breakdown of homeostasis

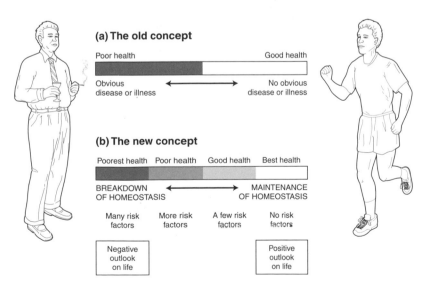

Figure 2.7 Nursing aspects of homeostasis: old and new concepts of health. Modified from Chiras D D, *Human Biology: Health, Homeostasis and the Environment*, 2nd edn, 1995 Boston: Jones & Bartlett Publishers. Reprinted with permission

while best health represents maintenance of homeostasis factors, no disease or illness and good fitness. Poorest health represents break-down of homeostasis while best health represents maintenance of homeostasis.

Thus where individuals are actively participating in measures that reduce many risk factors, such as stopping smoking, adopting a healthier diet by reducing fat and salt intake and eating more fresh fruit and vegetables, increasing exercise, adopting stress management measures that facilitate the reduction of stress, and monitoring own alcohol consumption level, they are actively facilitating homeostasis from a five-dimensional perspective. This perspective encompasses the physical, emotional, intellectual, social and spiritual aspects or dimen-sions of a person. The measures cited here boost an individual's self-esteem and help to create a positive outlook on life. Thus the stability of the internal environment is re-established both physiologically and emotionally.

Chiras' model (1995) supports the authors' view that health education and promotion aspects that health care workers reinforce with members of the public, especially at the primary care level such as in health care centres and other community venues, are very important in that not only does this identify risk in individuals but it also promotes homeostatic mechanisms in a way that involves consumers of health services as active participants rather than as passive recipients.

INFLUENCES OF THE EXTERNAL ENVIRONMENT ON HOMEOSTASIS

In recent years the importance of the external or global environment on health has been realised and has become more prominent. In Chapter 10 attention is given to the effect of stress on mental health. Environmental stresses related to noise, poor housing, poverty and homelessness do affect mental health and can produce demonstrable changes in normal biological processes. Not only are atmospheric pollut-ants implicated in the development and exacerbartion of pulmonary disease such as asthma, but they also can be the focus of anxiety and irrational thoughts leading to a disturbance of mental health. In order to illustrate some of the environmental concerns, a few examples are discussed here.

Great concern has been expressed about stratospheric ozone depletion and its potential damage to deoxyribonucleic acid (DNA) (Balmes 1991). The integrity of the ozone layer is vital to the protection of the genome of the vast majority of living organisms and, with regard to human health, ultraviolet (UV) light is strongly linked to the aetiology of skin cancers such as basal cell carcinoma, squamous cell carcinoma and cataracts

(Balmes 1991). The development of cancer is due to alteration of the internal environment as a result of internal and external challenges, the UV light being the initial external challenge.

Other external environmental challenges that may be of concern to public health are the long-term effects of chronic exposure to substances that include aluminium, lead, nitrates and pesticides which may be present in drinking water at low or very low concentrations. While the effects of aluminium on brain function and behaviour are still debatable, it has been implicated in arthritis, dementia and brittle bone disease (Seymour 1990). The effects of acute lead exposure are well established and include abdominal pain, headache, irritability and eventually coma and death (Walker 1992). Unfortunately, the effects of long-term low exposure are not yet fully known. There may be no neurotoxicity with some substances but there is no doubt that these substances do affect the stability of the internal environment.

Furthermore, in addition to what has just been described, the effects of air quality as an external challenge to the internal environment and to human health should not be underestimated since the oxides of nitrogen and petrochemical oxidants coupled with the mixture of the dioxides of nitrogen, sulphur and carbon are harmful (Read & Green 1990). While on the surface the effects of environmental pollution on the internal environment may appear to influence physical health most directly, the long-term effects of physical problems do have a significant bearing on the emotional well-being of individuals.

CONCLUSION

Homeostasis is not a static balance but a dynamic equilibrium in which continuous change occurs within the internal environment due to internal and external challenges and yet relatively uniform conditions prevail. This is achieved by feedback mechanisms that continually report the status of the internal environment to the control centre and by self-regulating processes that optimise conditions for survival. Nursing activity and interventions are about the promotion of physiological, emotional and spiritual well-being. When this is done this means that the stability of the internal environment has been achieved. Currently there is a missing link between an understanding of the concepts of homeostasis and nursing activity in different scenarios. This missing link results in failure to link theory to practice. As for homeostasis, Bernard reminded us over 100 years ago: 'a stable internal environment is the condition for free life' – life in which there are few or no risk factors to health.

REFERENCES

Antai-Otong D 1995 Stress, coping and adaptation. In: Antai-Otong D (ed) Psychiatric nursing: biological and behavioural concepts. Saunders, Philadelphia, p 119

Atkinson R L, Atkinson R C, Smith E E, Benn D J 1993 Introduction to psychology, 11th edn, Harcourt Brace College Publishers, Fort Worth, Texas

Balmes J R 1991 Propellant gases in metered dose inhalers: the impact on the global environment. Respiratory Care 36(9): 1037–1044

Benner P 1984 From novice to expert, excellence and power in clinical nursing practice. Addison Wesley, California

Cannon W B 1915 Bodily changes in pain hunger, fear and rage. Appleton, New York. Cited in: Best C H, Taylor N B 1937 The physiological basis of medical practice. Baillière, Tindall and Cox, London, P 1076–1098, 1593

Cannon W B 1932 The wisdom of the body. W W Norton, New York

Chiras D D 1995 Human biology: health, homeostasis and the environment, 2nd edn. West Publishing, St Paul, Minnesota

Clancy J, McVicar A 1994 Circadian rhythms 1: physiology. British Journal of Nursing 4(13): 657–661

Clancy J, McVicar A J 1995 Physiology and anatomy: a homeostatic approach. Edward Arnold, London

Colaizzi J 1975 The proper object of nursing science. International Journal of Nursing Studies 12: 197–200

David A S 1999 Auditory hallucinations: phenomenology, neuropsychology and neuroimaging update. Acta Psychiatrica Scandanavica 99 (suppl 395): 95–104

Dolan R J, Fletcher P C, McKenna P, Friston K J, Frith C D 1999 Abnormal neural integration related to cognition in schizophrenia. Acta Psychiatrica Scandanavica 99 (suppl 395): 58–67

Dunn A J 1995 Psychoneuroimmunology: introduction and general perspectives. In: Leonard B E, Miller K (eds) Stress, the immune system and psychiatry. John Wiley, Chichester, p 1–16

Egan G 1990 The skilled helper, a systematic approach to effective helping, 4th edn. Books/Cole Publishing Co., Pacific Grove, California

Encyclopaedia Britannica 1988a Bernard Claude. Micropaedia, vol 2, 15th edn. Encyclopaedia Britannica, Chicago

Encyclopaedia Britannica 1988b Cannon Walter Bradford. Micropaedia, vol 2, 15th edn, Encyclopaedia Britannica, Chicago

Ganong W F 1989 Review of medical physiology, 14th edn. Prentice-Hall, Connecticut

Hayes N 1994 Foundations of psychology an introductory text. Routledge, London

Hedlund N L, Jeffrey F B 1993 Overview of psychiatric nursing. In: Rawlins R P, Williams S R, Beck C K (eds) Mental health-psychiatric nursing: a holistic life-cycle approach, 3rd edn. Mosby Year Book, St Louis, p 2–16

Hilgard E R, Atkinson R L, Atkinson R C 1979 Introduction to psychology, 7th edn. Harcourt Brace Jovanovich, New York.

Hoffman R E 1999 New methods for studying hallucinated voices in schizophrenia. Acta Psychiatrica Scandanavica 99 (suppl 395): 89–94

Hole J W 1993 Human anatomy and physiology, 6th edn. Wm C. Brown, Dubuque, Iowa.

Hoover R M, Parnell P K 1984 An inpatient educational group on stress and coping. Journal of Psychosocial Nursing 22(6): 17–22

Kiecott-Glaser J K, Glaser R 1991 Stress and immune function in humans. In: Ader R, Felten D L, Cohen N (eds) Psychoneuroimmunology. Academic Press, San Diego, part IV, p 849–867

Menninger K 1963 The vital balance: the life process in mental health and illness. Viking Press, New York.

Pearson A, Vaughan B 1989 Nursing models in practice. Heinemann Nursing, Oxford

Peplau H E 1952 Interpersonal relations in nursing. G P Putnam, New York

Peplau H E 1988 Interpersonal relations in nursing. Macmillan Education, London

Read R, Green M 1990 Internal combustion and health. British Medical Journal 300: 761–762

Rinomhota A S, Cooper K 1996 Homeostasis: restoring the internal wellbeing in patients/clients. British Journal of Nursing 5(18): 1100–1108

Roberts M B V 1986 Biology: a functional approach, 4th edn. Nelson, Walton-on-Thames

Russell B 1989 Wisdom of the west: a historical survey of western philosophy in its social and political setting. Bloomsbury, London

Selye H 1974 Stress without distress. Lippincott, Philadelphia

Selye H 1976 The stress of life (review edn). McGraw-Hill, New York

Seymour J 1990 Water water everywhere. Nursing Times 86(44): 60–61

Sherwood L 1993 Human physiology – from cells to systems, 2nd edn. West Publishing, St Paul, Minnesota

Swanson K M 1991 Empirical development of a middle range theory of caring. Nursing Research 40(3): 161–166

Tudor E Mcl, Tudor E R 1985 Understanding the human body, 2nd edn. Pitman, Victoria, Australia

Tortora G J, Grabowski S R 1993 Principles of anatomy and physiology, 7th edn. Harper Collins, New York

Walker A 1992 Drinking water – doubts about quality. British Medical Journal 304: 175–178

Wilson-Barnett J, Batehup L 1988 Introduction: nursing knowledge, research and practice. In: Wilson-Barnett J, Batehup L Patient problems: a research base for nursing care. Scutari, London, p 1–7

3

Neuroanatomy and neurofunction

Many aspects of human behaviour and mental functioning can be better understood with some knowledge of the underlying biological processes.

(Atkinson et al, 1993, p 35)

In this chapter consideration is given to those aspects of the neuroanatomy and neurochemistry of the brain that seem most relevant to understanding altered thought, perception and behaviour associated with mental illness. In later chapters disordered neurophysiology is explored in relation to specific conditions and mental health problems. Within this chapter, most emphasis is given to the cerebral cortex, limbic system and closely connected structures, since the study of these regions has increased the understanding of behavioural changes in mental illness. The limbic system in particular has been implicated in the development of emotional disorders and current research is centred mainly around its activity.

ORGANISATION OF THE NERVOUS SYSTEM

Simplistically, the nervous system can be divided into two main parts, namely the *central nervous system* (CNS) and the *peripheral nervous system* (PNS). The CNS comprises of the brain and spinal cord while the PNS consists of sensory (afferent) and motor (efferent) nerves or neurones. The sensory neurones take information from different parts of the body to the brain and spinal cord for processing and integration. The motor neurones, on the other hand, take messages from the CNS to different organs, glands and muscles for execution of specific activities and responses. Some of these motor neurones convey voluntary information such as moving an arm or leg while others deal with autonomic (without voluntary control) responses. The autonomic part of the PNS has a sympathetic and a parasympathetic aspect, the details of which will be discussed later. Thus, the organisation of the nervous system can be illustrated diagramatically and very simply (Fig. 3.1)

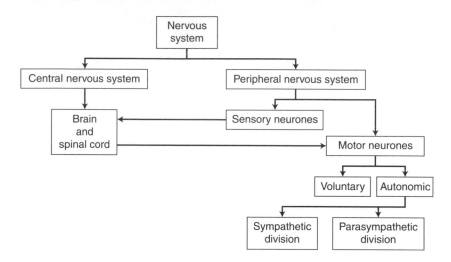

Figure 3.1   The organisation of the nervous system.

THE CENTRAL NERVOUS SYSTEM

The brain of an average adult weighs about 1300 g and is made up of about 100 billion neurones and 900 billion neuroglial cells. The structures that form the mature brain can be described in various ways. From an embryological perspective, the mature adult brain develops from five dilatations which are established by the time the embryo is at six weeks of gestation. These dilatations are classified as:

- telencephalon
- diencephalon
- mesencephalon
- metencephalon
- myelencephalon.

These five dilatations undergo major growth and develop into the three major gross parts classified in the adult mature brain as the cerebrum, cerebellum and brainstem (Fig. 3.2). The brainstem is further subdivided into:

- midbrain (the uppermost part)
- pons (the middle region)
- medulla oblongata (the lowest part of the brainstem).

The major portion of the cerebrum develops from the telencephalon, the thalamus and hypothalamus from the diencephalon, the midbrain from the mesencephalon, the cerebellum and pons from the metencephalon and the medulla oblongata from the myelencephalon.

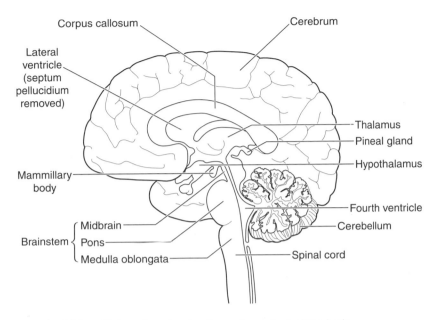

Figure 3.2 Mid-sagittal section showing the major regions of the brain.

THE CEREBRUM AND CEREBRAL CORTEX

The cerebrum consists of the left and right cerebral hemispheres, incompletely separated by the deep longitudinal fissure. The surface of the cerebrum is composed of a layer of grey matter, 1.3–4.5 mm in thickness, which is referred to as the cerebral cortex. Despite its relative thinness, the cerebral cortex is highly complex, is composed of six well-differentiated layers of nerve cell bodies arranged in columns and is estimated to contain around 14 billion nerve cells (Gilman & Newman 1996).

Furthermore, during embryonic development, the grey matter enlarges out of proportion to the underlying white matter. As a consequence the cerebral cortex folds upon itself to form the characteristic features of the cortex which include convolutions (gyri), the large and deep grooves (fissures) and the less deep grooves (sulci).

For descriptive purposes the lateral surfaces of the cerebral hemispheres have been divided into four lobes (Fig. 3.3A):

- frontal
- parietal
- temporal
- occipital.

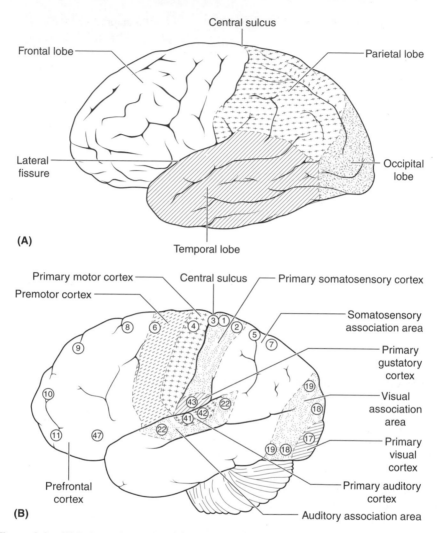

Figure 3.3 (A) Lobes of the cerebral cortex. (B) Selected functional areas of the cerebral cortex. The numbers indicate specific brain regions as plotted by Brodmann (1909).

A fifth lobe, the *insula*, lies deep within the lateral cerebral fissure, under the parietal, frontal and temporal lobes (Gilman & Newman, 1996).

Furthermore, specific areas of the cortex have been identified, as described by Brodmann (1909), who first published a cytoarchitectural map of the cortex as an attempt to correlate structure with function. Figure 3.3B provides a simplified view of the functional areas of the cortex, with the most important Brodmann areas numbered.

It is now understood that the specific columnar arrangement of the neurones in the cortex has important functional significance. It seems that cortical neurones form connections within columns and also between adjacent columns thus allowing for an amplifying effect on nerve impulses, for example, permitting sufficient motor neurones to discharge for movement and, in the sensory cortex, to distinguish two closely related stimuli (Trimble 1996). Broadly, the cortex can be divided functionally into three areas:

- sensory
- motor
- association.

Sensory function

As stated earlier, the sensory neurones are involved in conveying information from peripheral receptors to the CNS and are concerned with making sense of changes in the external and internal (the fluid surrounding the cells) environment. Each sensory neurone has a specific *receptive field*. Neurones may connect to several receptors over a given area on the body surface. Stimulation of any of the receptors will generate impulses in the same sensory neurone. The area covered by the sensory neurone is called the receptive field. It is very specific for each neurone and varies considerably between neurones.

Somatosensory cortex

General senses (somatic) include cutaneous sensations, the sensations of temperature, pressure, touch and pain and are interpreted in the anterior portions of the parietal lobes called the primary somatosensory cortex (Fig. 3.3B). It lies along the central sulcus, in a region described as the postcentral gyrus, and the cell bodies found in the somatosensory cortex are arranged in columns. The location of the columns of cell bodies is related systematically to the location of the receptive fields on the body surface and the columns are organised in such a way as to create a somatic sensory map (Gilman & Newman 1996).

Afferent fibres from receptors located in specific parts of the body terminate in specific regions of the sensory cortex thus presenting a sensory map. The sensory map in humans is called a homunculus, meaning 'little man'. Figure 3.4A is a diagramatic representation of the homunculus. As can be seen, the cell bodies in the cortex on the lateral surface of the somatosensory cortex, just above the lateral fissure, have receptive fields on the face and, as another example, cell bodies on the more superior part of the cortex have receptive fields on the hands and

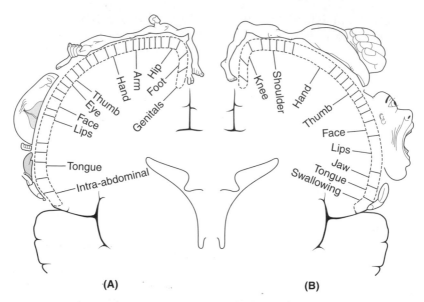

Figure 3.4 (A) Sensory homunculus. (B) Motor homunculus.

arms. Furthermore, regions of the body such as the face and hands have a proportionally larger number of receptors, and therefore a larger receptive field, so these regions take up a larger proportion of the map.

The somatosensory cortex is responsible for the processing of somatosensory information. However, it also appears to have higher-order processing abilities, such as the recognition of special features of a stimulus, leading to discrimination in the intensity and direction of the applied stimulus as well as the location (Berne & Levy 1996).

Motor function

Motor function involves several areas of the cerebral hemispheres. However two areas are of primary importance:

- Primary motor cortex
- Premotor area.

Primary motor cortex

The primary motor cortex of each cerebral hemisphere lies in the frontal lobes, anterior to the central sulcus (precentral gyrus) as shown in Figure 3.3B. The nervous tissue in these regions contains numerous large pyramid-shaped cell bodies. Impulses from these pyramidal cells are conducted downward through the brainstem and into the spinal cord. As with the sensory cortex, the motor cortex is also organised to create a map of the body based on the number of motor neurones associated with a particular region of the body and can be represented in the form of a motor homunculus (Fig. 3.4B). The parts of the body capable of delicate or fine movement (e.g. fingers and lips) have a large cortical representation, whereas those performing relatively gross movements (e.g. trunk and shoulders) have a small representation.

The nerve cells in the primary motor cortex are organised into columns which extend vertically from the surface into the deeper layers of the cortex. A single column is a functional entity responsible for directing a specific group of muscles acting on a single joint. In general the primary motor cortex is the region through which commands are channelled for the execution of specific movements (Barr & Kiernan 1993). Lesions in the primary motor cortex result immediately in varying degrees of paresis of the muscles of the opposite side of the body (hemiparesis and hemiplegia), with hypotonia (decreased resistance to passive manipulation) and decreased muscle stretch reflexes.

Premotor area

The premotor area (Brodmann area 6, Fig. 3.3B) lies in front of the primary motor cortex, on the lateral surface of the cerebral hemisphere and, along with other areas in the cortex, such as the supplementary motor area, the second motor area and secondary somatic sensory area (located in the parietal lobe), is involved in controlling the proper sequence of voluntary movement (Barr & Kiernan 1993, Carpenter 1996, Noback et al 1996). The premotor cortex has a primary role in the control of proximal limb and axial musculature and is essential for the initial orientation movements of the body, for example positioning the body before playing a tennis stroke (Noback et al 1996).

The supplementary motor area, which lies medially to the premotor area, seems to have a role in the programming of patterns and sequences of movements (Barr & Kiernan 1993, Carpenter 1996, Noback et al 1996). It is also thought to be involved in the advanced planning of movements, particularly for movements involving both sides of the body (Gilman & Newman 1996). The second motor area and secondary somatic sensory area are both located at the base of the pre- and postcentral gyrus, but their functional significance is not fully understood. Collectively the premotor cortex and supplementary areas are involved in the control of skilled motor activity and direct the primary motor area in the execution of these activities. Lesions in the premotor area result in different forms of apraxia, which can be defined as the impairment in performance of learned motor activities in the absence of paralysis.

Association areas

Association areas are those areas of the cerebrum that are interconnected with sensory and motor areas and with other areas of the brain. These areas occupy the anterior regions of the frontal lobes (prefrontal cortex) and are widespread in the lateral portions of the parietal, temporal and occipital lobes. It is suggested that association areas are involved in the analysis and interpretation of sensory experiences as well as reasoning, memory and emotional responses (Gilman & Newman 1996). The prefrontal cortex also seems to play a part in mood and emotional experience and, as will be discussed later in this chapter, it is closely linked to the limbic system.

CEREBRUM: WHITE MATTER

Underlying the cortex is a complex array of white matter, consisting of myelinated axons, which are classified as:

- association fibres
- commissural fibres
- projection fibres.

Some fibres serve to link areas in the same hemisphere (association fibres) while other fibres link areas in one hemisphere to the same areas in the opposite hemisphere (commissural fibres). Projection fibres link the cerebrum to other parts of the brain and spinal cord via ascending and descending fibres. The association fibres are the most numerous and the corpus callosum forms the largest collection of commissural fibres.

CEREBRUM: INTERNAL GREY MATTER STRUCTURES

There are several important areas of grey matter that lie deep within the cerebrum which are involved in sensory perception, thought, emotional experience and behaviour. Some of these areas include the thalamus, hypothalamus, basal ganglia and limbic system.

Thalamus

The thalamus is generally considered to play a pivotal role in the transmission of somatic sensory impulses to the cerebral cortex. It is a dumbbell-shaped mass of grey matter situated just above the hypothalamus and is subdivided into three main groups of cell bodies, classified as:

- medial nuclear masses
- lateral nuclear masses
- anterior thalamic nucleus.

Afferent nerve impulses are received from the spinal cord via, for example, the spinothalamic tracts, from the basal ganglia, the cerebellum, the reticular formation located in the brainstem and various parts of the cerebrum. The thalamus also has connections with the frontal lobes, particularly the prefrontal cortex and the limbic system, as well as widespread connections throughout the somatosensory cortex, so that virtually all areas of the cortex receive nerve impulses from the thalamus.

From a functional perspective, the thalamus is involved in the recognition of crude sensations of pain, touch and temperature. It also seems that the thalamus plays a part in the emotional component linked to sensory interpretation through the association of sensory impulses with the feelings of pleasantness or unpleasantness. It also has a further role in memory. In essence the thalamus serves as a relay station (the sensory switchboard), from which, after processing, nerve impulses from all types of sensory receptors are directed on to the cerebral cortex.

Hypothalamus

The hypothalamus consists of several structures that lie beneath the thalamus and above the pituitary gland and form the floor of the third ventricle. The arrangement of the hypothalamus is very complex. From anatomical and neurophysiological perspectives, the hypothalamus has been described in terms of various zones and regions and in terms of specific groups of cell bodies. The specific groups of cell bodies are sometimes identified as hypothalamic nuclei and hypothalamic areas.

To simplify matters, Table 3.1 provides a list of the four regions generally described with the groups of cell bodies broadly located within each region.

Table 3.1 Organisation of the hypothalamus

Region	Main hypothalamic areas/nuclei
Preoptic region	
Anterior hypothalamic region (supraoptic area)	Suprachiasmatic nuclei Supraoptic nuclei Paraventricular nuclei Anterior hypothalamic area Lateral hypothalamic area
Tuberal region	Ventromedial nucleus Dorsomedial nucleus Arcuate nucleus
Mamillary region	Mamillary bodies Posterior hypothalamic area

Table 3.2 Some of the major functions of the hypothalamus

Regions and nuclei of hypothalamus	Functions
Supraoptic and paraventricular nuclei	Synthesis and secretion of antidiuretic hormone (ADH) and oxytocin Role in producing circadian rhythms in animals
Arcuate nucleus	Secrete hypothalamic releasing/inhibiting factors
Ventromedial nucleus and lateral hypothalamic area	Role in control of autonomic nervous system Role in control of feeding and body weight Role in control of emotional state in animals
Mamillary bodies	Role in memory Role in control of limbic system outflow and emotions
Preoptic region, anterior hypothalamic area and posterior hypothalamic area	Body temperature regulation
Preoptic region, anterior hypothalamic area, ventromedial nucleus and arcuate nucleus	Regulation of sexual behaviour and gonadal function

The preoptic area is histologically indistinguishable from the hypothalamus and functionally inseparable from the anterior hypothalamus, so most authorities include it with the hypothalamus.

Although the hypothalamus is small, it has a functional importance quite out of proportion to its size and is an important site for much of the convergence of the limbic system. While discrete groups of cell bodies can be identified in the human hypothalamus, based on the limited current understanding of the specific functions of each group, a more generalised view of the function of the hypothalamus has to be taken. Table 3.2 provides a list of some of the main functions of the hypothalamus.

First, the hypothalamus is directly involved in regulating autonomic nervous system activity. The hypothalamus functions as several higher autonomic centres, with connections to parasympathetic and sympathetic centres in the brainstem and spinal cord. As such it is involved in the control and integration of autonomic responses throughout the body. Furthermore, the hypothalamus functions as an important relay station between the cerebral cortex and lower autonomic centres, thus linking the *psyche* and the *soma*.

The paraventricular and supraoptic region of the hypothalamus is essentially involved in neuroendocrine activity. The axons from neurones in these areas are neurosecretory fibres connected to the posterior pituitary gland. The hormones antidiuretic hormone (vasopressin) and oxytocin are synthesised in the paraventricular and supraoptic nuclei and transported for storage to the posterior pituitary gland (neurohypophysis) via the neurosecretory axons. Other hypothalamic nuclei synthesise and secrete neuropeptides which act as regulating hormones and modify the release of hormones from the anterior pituitary gland (adenohypophysis). For example, the release of adrenocorticotrophic hormone (ACTH), which is involved in the response to stress, is governed by the regulating hormone produced by the hypothalamus called corticotrophin releasing hormone (CRH; Thibodeau & Patton 1993).

The hypothalamus is further involved in the regulation of body temperature, the regulation of thirst and appetite and in maintaining the waking state. It also exhibits properties of a self-sustained oscillator and as such drives many biological rhythms (Trimble 1996).

Basal ganglia

The basal ganglia are masses of interconnected grey matter located deep within the cerebral hemispheres. From a clinical and physiological perspective, the term basal ganglia refers collectively to the following structures:

- corpus striatum
- subthalamic nucleus
- substantia nigra.

The corpus striatum is a substantial mass of grey matter near the base of each cerebral hemisphere. The corpus striatum is further composed of specific nuclei, as follows:

Corpus striatum   =   caudate nucleus
                        +
                        lentiform nucleus   =   putamen
                                                  +
                                                  globus pallidus

The substantia nigra is a large nucleus located in the midbrain. It is composed of the pars compacta and the pars reticulata. It seems to influence the activity of the striatum (the caudate nucleus and putamen). Fibres that arise in the pars compacta and synapse in the striatum use the neurotransmitter dopamine.

Mapping of the circuitry shows that the basal ganglia interact with the cerebral cortex through a series of feedback circuits. As such the basal ganglia, along with the cerebellum, are influenced by and influence the motor cortex and other parts of the cortex that give rise to the descending motor pathways. Experimental studies on animals (Kötter & Meyer 1992) suggest that the basal ganglia monitor the progress of movements and have a major role in the automatic execution of learned motor activity. Take the example of subconsciously swinging one's arms when walking: this is due to the activity of the basal ganglia.

Lesions that occur in the basal ganglia in humans result in a number of movement disorders, including disorders in the initiation of movement (akinesia), difficulty stopping movement, abnormalities of muscle tone and the development of involuntary movement (e.g. tremor). Parkinson's disease is an example of a condition arising from a disorder of the basal ganglia. It is associated with neuronal degeneration of the pars compacta region of the substantia nigra, resulting in a depletion of dopamine and complex changes in the activity of projection neurones between the substantia nigra and the striatum. The movement problems encountered by individuals who suffer from Parkinson's disease include akinesia, muscle rigidity and tremor.

Limbic system

Due to the increasing importance of the limbic system in the understanding of feelings and behaviour, this area of the brain is discussed in more detail. Trimble (1996) provides a historical overview. Willis (1664) referred to an area of the brain around the brainstem as the *cerebri limbus*, while Broca (1878) defined a comparative but more extensive area as *'le grand lobe limbique'*. It seems that it was not until the middle of the 20th century that the concept of the limbic system was developed and a link with the emotions was identified (Maclean 1970, Papez 1937).

As a general statement the limbic system is a wishbone-shaped group of structures that encircles the brainstem and is involved in both the objective expression and the subjective experience of emotions. The name *limbic* (Latin for 'border or fringe') provides some idea as to the shape of the structures that make up the limbic system. Essentially, part of the limbic structures form a curving border following the line of the corpus callosum.

In the literature there appears to be some variation in the structures that are described as forming the limbic system. Nauta & Domesick (1982) provide a discussion on the various structures although, generally speaking, there are some structures that are common to all the literature (Fig. 3.5, Table 3.3). Any definition of the limbic system stresses the link to the hypothalamus and includes the hypocampus, amygdala, some regions of the thalamus, parts of the temporal lobe and parts of the basal ganglia.

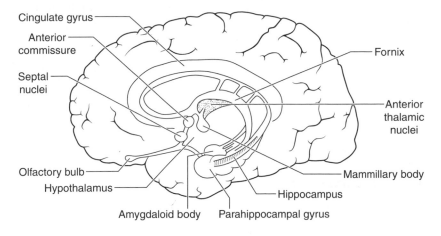

Figure 3.5 Selected components of the limbic system and associated structures.

Table 3.3 Major components of the limbic system

Component	Anatomical region
Areas of cortex	Cingulate gyrus Parahippocampal gyrus Septal area Temporal lobe (temporal neocortex and entorhinal cortex)
Nuclei	Amygdala Anterior thalamic nuclei Hippocampal formation Hypothalamus Mamillary body
Fibres/pathways	Fornix

In recent studies relying upon extremely sophisticated techniques employing immunohistochemistry, Niewenhuys (1996) has identified additional connections involving ultra-thin nerve fibres, to groups of neurones in the pons and medulla, which seem to be involved in autonomic and somatomotor integration. Niewenhuys (1996) describes this as the greater limbic system.

Many different neurotransmitters have been identified in the limbic system; all emphasising the complex nature and function of the limbic system. Gamma-amino butyric acid (GABA) is an important inhibitory transmitter located in the amygdala and hippocampus. However, acetylcholine, histamine, noradrenaline, serotonin and dopamine are all found in various concentrations throughout the different structures forming the limbic system (Ben-Ari 1981, Roberts et al 1984).

The limbic system as a whole seems to be involved in the discrimination of stimuli in terms of their behavioural significance and the storing of these stimuli in the short-term memory (Barker 1991). It is fundamentally involved in controlling emotional responses to stimuli and the expression of emotional responses through the autonomic nervous system.

THE AUTONOMIC NERVOUS SYSTEM

The autonomic nervous system is the entire mass of those nerve cells and fibres involved in the stimulation and regulation of internal organs and glands. It is essentially involved in the involuntary control of organ function and, as discussed in Chapter 2, the maintenance of homeostasis through the regulation of the internal environment. As with the somatic (voluntary) nervous system the autonomic nervous system has both sensory and motor components. The motor component consists of two divisions:

- sympathetic
- parasympathetic.

Both are anatomically distinct, they use different neurotransmitters at the target gland or organ synapse where they activate different receptors and in many cases exert opposing effects. Both systems have ganglia which are collections of cell bodies. Axons run from the spinal cord to the ganglia and are known as preganglionic fibres while other axons run from the ganglia to effectors which may be muscle, organ or gland, where they effect changes. The latter are known as postganglionic fibres.

Sympathetic nervous system

The nerves involved in this division leave a region of the spinal cord extending from the thoracic segment to the upper lumbar area (spinal cord levels T1–L2). For this reason the sympathetic nervous system is described as the thoracolumbar system. Most of the ganglia of the sympathetic division lie either side of and close to the spinal cord, arranged as a chain. Hence this division has short preganglionic fibres and long postganglionic fibres. Also, importantly, the chain of ganglia are all interconnected and therefore the sympathetic nervous system activates many effectors simultaneously, thus *producing a whole body response.*

With regard to the neurochemistry, the major neurotransmitters involved at the endings of postganglionic fibres are noradrenaline and adrenaline. Noradrenaline is chiefly synthesised and released from the axon ending, while adrenaline is mainly secreted from the adrenal medulla, to augment the sympathetic effects. For this reason, sympathetic nerve fibres are also described as *adrenergic fibres.* At least four different receptors located on the target cells have been identified to which nora-drenaline and adrenaline bind to produce the physiological effects. The receptors are classified as α and β receptors, each with particular sub-types:

- α_1 and α_2
- β_1, β_2 and β_3.

Different tissues and cells possess more of one type of receptor than the other, thus allowing for a variety of differing effects to occur in different tissues and organs. Noradrenaline and adrenaline both act on α and β receptors. However, noradrenaline tends to have a stronger action on α receptors, whereas adrenaline has a stronger action on β receptors.

Parasympathetic nervous system

The parasympathetic division consists of the cranial nerves III, VII, IX and X (vagus) and the sacral nerves (S2–S4). For this reason the parasympathetic division is often called the craniosacral system. Unlike the sympathetic system, the parasympathetic ganglia lie distant from the spinal cord, being located near to or within the effec-tor cells/organs. Thus the parasympathetic division has long pregan-glionic fibres and short postganglionic fibres. More importantly, the ganglia are not interconnected, so unlike the sympathetic division, the parasympathetic system *does not produce an integrated, whole body response.* Different tissues tend to be activated individually, for example gastric activity can be stimulated (via the vagus nerve) without the heart rate becoming slower (also mediated through branches of the vagus nerve).

The parasympathetic division is also described as cholinergic since the major neurotransmitter involved in the activity of this division is acetylcholine and the receptors to which acetylcholine binds are classed as cholinergic receptors. Subtypes of these receptors also exist:

- nicotinic (found at ganglionic synapse)
- muscarinic (found on target cells).

Overall functions of the autonomic nervous system

The major function of the sympathetic system is to produce a series of responses to deal with 'stress' and increased physical activity. Collectively these responses increase the availability and utilisation of energy. It was Walter B. Cannon (1930) who coined the now-familiar phrase *fight-or-flight reaction*, to describe the function and action of the sympathetic nervous system. The key words to describe sympathetic activity are acceleration and mobilisation for activity. On the other hand, during quiet, non-stressful conditions, it is the parasympathetic division that is dominant. The parasympathetic nervous system is concerned with restoration and the conservation of energy. The key words are braking, relaxation and recuperation.

The autonomic nervous system as a whole functions to maintain or quickly restore homeostasis. Most organs and tissues are innervated by the sympathetic and parasympathetic divisions and thus have *dual innervation*. Both divisions continually conduct nerve impulses to the effector tissues and organs and both are said to be *tonically active*. As they tend to produce opposite effects, the overall effect of the autonomic nervous system on a given organ depends upon the balance in activity between the two divisions. For example, the sympathetic division tends to increase the heart rate while the parasympathetic division slows it down. The actual heart rate therefore depends upon which division is most active.

Another important point to understand is that the autonomic nervous system is also influenced by the higher centres of the brain. As identified earlier, the autonomic nervous system is modified by the nerve impulses from the frontal cortex, limbic system and the hypothalamus.

Biofeedback

Individuals can learn to control specific autonomic activities (e.g. heart rate and blood pressure) if they are informed that they are achieving the desired response (e.g. a reduction in heart rate and lowering of blood pressure). Various biofeedback instruments have been developed to provide the required feedback and biofeedback as a technique has been used in the management of obsessive–compulsive disorders and panic attacks.

The ability of an individual to interpret stimuli, make sense of her environment and respond appropriately requires the integrated transmission of information throughout all areas of the nervous system. This process involves sensory and motor neurones (Fig. 3.6) and it is important to consider how information is transmitted and processed. In simple terms, information is transmitted as a nerve impulse.

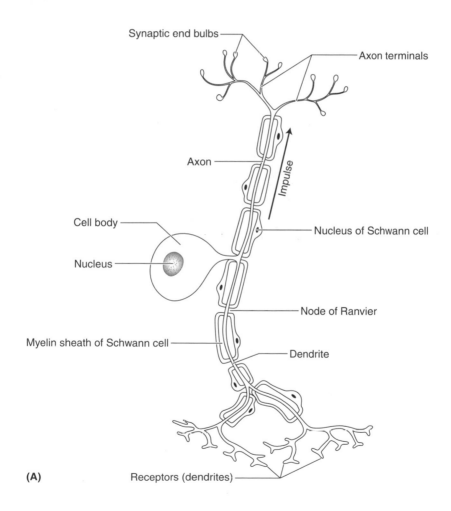

Figure 3.6 (A) Peripheral sensory (afferent) neurone: myelinated.

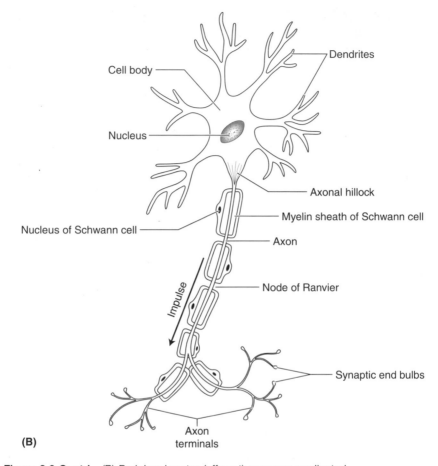

Figure 3.6 Contd   (B) Peripheral motor (efferent) neurone: myelinated.

NEUROTRANSMITTERS AND THE NERVE IMPULSE

The nerve impulse

All excitable cells have a resting membrane potential whose magnitude varies from tissue to tissue (Ganong 1999, Hille 1992). In a nerve cell at rest, the inside of its membrane is negatively charged while the outside is positively charged. Since potassium and magnesium are intracellular ions while sodium and calcium are extracellular ions, this means that the inside of the nerve cell membrane is high in potassium ions (K^+) and the outside is high in sodium ions (Na^+). Electrical potentials are generated by the passive movement of ions such as Na^+, K^+, Ca^{++},

Mg^{++} and Cl^- through highly selective molecular pores in the cell surface membrane called ionic channels. Ionic channels play an important role in membrane excitation and the opening and closing of specific pores gives rise to characteristic electrical messages. Signals that make the cytoplasm more positive are said to depolarize the membrane, and those that make it more negative are said to hyperpolarize the membrane.

Each cell has a point above which a stimulus will produce an action potential and below which an action potential will not occur. This point is called the threshold potential. Therefore in order for a cell to be excited and for an action potential to be produced, the cell must receive a stimulus that is strong enough to reach the threshold potential. Once the threshold has been reached the action potential will be generated.

The action potential results from a number of events summarised in Table 3.4. When an excitatory stimulus strong enough to reach the threshold is applied, a rapid movement of sodium ions into the cell by diffusion occurs. This is due to the opening of sodium ion channels which are voltage sensitive. These channels are sometimes referred to as voltage-gated channels (Ganong 1999, Llinas 1988). The result of this influx of sodium ions is to make the inside of the cell more positive (depolarisation). In fact the voltage inside the nerve cell changes from $-70 \, mV$ to $+30 \, mV$.

The reversal of these events occurs as the inside of the cell becomes more positive. This is called repolarisation and occurs due to the opening

Table 3.4   Events of nerve cell in resting state and under nerve impulse activation

Nerve state	Cell membrane activity
Nerve cell in resting state	No nerve impulse is transmitted Sodium (Na^+) channel closed Potassium (K^+) channels closed Na^+/K^+ pump maintains ionic imbalance of cell membrane More Na^+ ions outside nerve cell membrane More K^+ ions inside nerve cell membrane
Nerve cell in activated state	Difference in potential (voltage) across cell Sodium channels open first and allow sodium ions to enter nerve cell membrane Shortly afterwards sodium channels close and potassium ions open Potassium ions move out of nerve cell membrane Potassium channels close Sequence of events carries nerve impulse forward

of voltage-sensitive potassium ion channels. This occurs as the voltage-sensitive sodium channels close thus preventing sodium from entering the cell. The net effect is for potassium ions to diffuse out of the cell making the inside of the cell membrane more negative again compared to the outer surface of the membrane. Eventually the normal resting membrane potential is restored as the NA^+-K^+ pump located in the cell membrane restores the normal distribution of sodium and potassium both within and outside the cell.

In short, an action potential is a brief, spike-like depolarisation that propagates regeneratively as an electrical wave without decrement and at a high, constant velocity from one end of the axon to the other. Once the action potential has been generated, it moves along the axon of the nerve cell as an impulse.

Depolarisation is a momentary event since both ions are quickly returned to their respective parts of the membrane by a sodium–potassium pump. The production and transmission of an action potential occurs in both afferent and efferent neurones. Table 3.4 gives a summary of the events describing the nerve impulse.

A nerve is a bundle of nerve fibres (neurones) in the PNS or CNS. Some nerves are made up of sensory neurones and others are made up of motor neurones. Most nerves have both sensory and motor neurones and are therefore known as mixed nerves. It is important to note here that often when people are not feeling well emotionally, they sometimes describe themselves as 'suffering from nerves'. Implicit in this phrase is the ability of individuals to notice that their thinking, their feelings (or emotions) and their behaviour are different from when they are well. It is therefore necessary for practitioners to understand how information is passed from one neurone to another.

The synapse

The term *synapse* was first introduced in 1897 by Sherrington to refer to special locus of contact between two neurones (De Robertis 1964), to describe the hypothetical region specialised for the exchange of signals between cells (Hucho 1986) and to mean the junction between two neurones. A synapse is a connection that is made when an axon ends nearer another cell. This connection is functional. Synapses occur between two neurones and between a neurone and muscle tissue. When the axon of one neurone connects with either the dendrites or cell body (Fig. 3.7), a neurone–neurone connection is formed. A tiny gap known as a synaptic cleft is found in the synapse (Fig. 3.8). The communication that occurs between two neurones or between a neurone and muscle at the synapse is not electrical but chemical. The chemicals that make this communication possible are known as neurotransmitters.

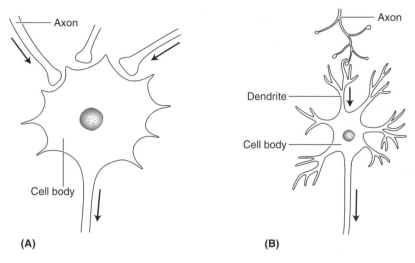

Figure 3.7   Synapse arrangement. (A) Axon to cell body. (B) Axon to dendrites.

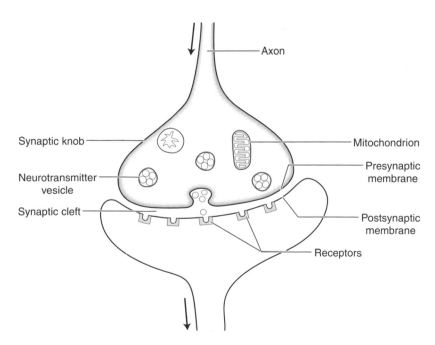

Figure 3.8   The synapse.

Neurotransmitters

To put things into perspective, an understanding of neurotransmitters and how they work is an asset for mental health nurses, since drugs that act on the CNS are used more widely, all over the world, than any other type of drug (Neal 1997). Two additional factors that need to be considered by mental health nurses are the sense of well-being that is produced by the therapeutic use of agents that include alcohol, caffeine and nicotine coupled with the dependence and addiction produced by the same agents as well as by the controlled drugs.

The logical questions to ask are: what are neurotransmitters? Where do they come from? How and where do they work? What do they actually do in the body?

Historical perspective

An interesting and detailed history of the discovery of neurotransmitters is given by Hucho (1986) while a detailed summary of the properties of the main CNS neurotransmitters is given by Hucho (1986), Siegel et al (1996), Barker (1991) and Gilman & Newman (1996). As far back as 1877, Du Bois Reymond suggested that it was possible for the presynaptic cell to influence the postsynaptic cell either by electrical currents or by chemical mediators (Siegel et al 1996). This was followed by the chemical transmission theory (Elliot 1904 cited in De Robertis 1964), which implies that a 'chemical mechanism is interposed at the junction between two components of the synapse' (De Robertis 1964). Elliot's suggestion was that sympathetic nerves acted by releasing adrenaline at their junctional regions with smooth muscles. Two years later Dixon (1906 cited in Hucho 1986) proposed that parasympathetic nerves acted by releasing a substance similar to muscarine.

It is now established that noradrenaline is the real sympathetic transmitter. Work by Dale in 1914 demonstrated the inhibitory effects of acetylcholine on heart muscle and strongly supported the chemical transmitter hypothesis by Loewi in 1921 (Loewi 1935) who found that stimulation of the vagus nerve reduced the heartbeat. Cannon (1930) suggested that the sympathetic nervous system had an emergency mechanism brought into action under conditions of 'fright, fight or flight', the so-called 'sympathetic discharge'. Soon afterwards, acetylcholine release from sympathetic ganglia was demonstrated by Feldberg & Gaddum in 1934 and from skeletal muscles in 1935 by Dale, and by Feldberg & Voigt in 1948.

In 1955 Von Euler established that noradrenaline is the sympathetic neurotransmitter and not adrenaline (De Robertis 1964) while Curtis and Watkins (1960) found that glutamic, aspartic and cysteic acids cause excitation of spinal interneurones and motorneurones. More recently, Krnjevic (1974) noticed that some brain cells are excited by 5–hydroxytryptamine (5HT) while others are inhibited by it.

Thus the history of neurotransmitters demonstrates not only the tremendous amount of work that has gone on in order to try and understand the role of neurotransmitters, but also the need for more understanding of these neurotransmitters in terms of how they influence brain function.

The nature and origin of neurotransmitters

Neurotransmitters are chemical substances that are synthesised in the nervous system. The protein in food that individuals consume is broken down to simpler molecules called amino acids. These amino acids become the starting point or precursors in the synthesis of some of the neurotransmitters. Table 3.5 summarises some of the neurotransmitters, their precursor amino acids and their effect.

In general neurotransmitters produce their action at receptors by two different mechanisms and it is the nature of the receptors that determine the mechanism (Gilman & Newman 1996). At some receptors known as *ionotropic receptors*, some neurotransmitters are able to alter the state of ionic channels in the postsynaptic membrane (Fig. 3.8), resulting in a rapid or quick response. An example of such a neurotransmitter is 5-hydroxytryptamine (5HT). Other neurotransmitters act at *G-protein coupled receptors* by a cascade of reactions that change the metabolism of the postsynaptic cell via second messengers. Examples of such neurotransmitters are dopamine, adrenaline and noradrenaline.

Second messengers are chemicals involved in reactions or processes in an indirect manner but are so important that, when missing, the reaction or process will not occur. The first messenger molecule (e.g. the neurotransmitter molecule) interacts with a membrane-bound receptor

Table 3.5 Neurotransmitters and their precursor amino acids

Precursor amino acid	Neurotransmitter	Role (example)
Choline	Acetylcholine	Memory and cognition
Tyrosine	Dopamine	
	Noradrenaline (norepinephrine)	Alertness
	Adrenaline (epinephrine)	
Tryptophan	Serotonin (5-hydroxytryptamine, 5HT)	Calmness
Glutamic acid	Gamma aminobutyric acid (GABA)	Damps down CNS excitablility and neuronal responsiveness

molecule. The second messenger then acts as a signal and carries information to a site within the cell. Examples of second messengers are cyclic adenosine monophosphate (cyclic AMP), cyclic guanosine monophosphate (cyclic GMP), diacylglycerol (DAG) and inositol triphosphate (IP$_3$). The neurotransmitters that act at G-protein coupled receptors produce longer lasting effects due to the cascade nature of the process and include dopamine, noradrenaline, adrenaline and neuropeptides (Gilman & Newman 1996). Gamma amino butyric acid (GABA), glutamic acid, aspartic acid and acetylcholine have an effect on inotropic and G-protein coupled receptors (Gilman & Newman 1996).

Neurotransmitters are required for the transmission of nerve impulses across the synapses (Fig. 3.8). Each neurotransmitter is released from the vesicle holding it (neurotransmitter vesicle) when an impulse arrives at the synapse. Calcium ions enter the synaptic vesicle and this causes the synaptic vesicle to fuse with the presynaptic membrane and release the neurotransmitter into the synaptic cleft. On its release from the vesicle, the neurotransmitter crosses the synaptic gap or cleft by diffusion and attaches itself to a receptor molecule that is consistent with its own shape like a 'lock and key'. A new action potential, the message, is generated and the message continues on its voyage. Some neurotransmitters excite the next neurone while others inhibit it. An excitatory neurotransmitter is one that causes the postsynaptic neurone more likely to fire action potentials, and an inhibitory neurotransmitter is one that makes the postsynaptic neurone less likely to fire action potentials. An example of an excitatory neurotransmitter is glutamic acid which is found in the brain, and an example of an inhibitory neurotransmitter is GABA.

Acetylcholine

Acetylcholine was first identified as a possible mediator of cellular function by Hunt in 1907 while in 1914, Dale highlighted the similarities in acetylcholine action with the response of the parasympathetic nervous system (Taylor & Brown, 1989). Clear evidence that acetylcholine was released by nerve stimulation was provided by Loewi in 1921 (Taylor & Brown 1989).

Acetylcholine is found in many different organisms including bacteria, fungi and protozoa as well as plants. In mammals acetylcholine can be found in high concentrations in sites where it has no known function such as the cornea, ciliated epithelia, the spleen of some ungulates (animals that chew the cud) and the placenta (Taylor & Brown 1989). In humans acetylcholine is synthesised, stored and released by preganglionic autonomic neurones and postganglionic parasympathetic neurones (Trimble 1996). It is distributed throughout the CNS as well as outside it with high concentrations of the neurotransmitter being found in the cerebral cortex, thalamus and several nuclei. Acetylcholine is also released at neuromuscular junctions of cardiac muscle, smooth muscles and skeletal muscles and its role in cholinergic transmission is well known (Purves et al 1997). However, while acetylcholine is one of the most studied neurotransmitters, it must be stated here that its role in the CNS is not yet clearly understood (Purves et al 1997).

MacIntosh (1981) suggests that acetylcholine synthesis in the brain may be limited by the availability of choline and cites work by Haubrich & Chippendale (1977) and Ulus et al (1978) who showed that brain acetylcholine level rises significantly when plasma choline is increased. Observations have shown that while ganglia and muscles can maintain their acetylcholine stores in an almost undiminished state even during intense synaptic activity, the cortex acetylcholine stores are always in a state of partial depletion (Tucek et al 1990).

There are two types of acetylcholine receptor. One type is stimulated by nicotine, a drug found in tobacco leaves, while the other type is stimulated by muscarine, a drug found in a poisonous mushroom. The receptor stimulated by nicotine is known as the nicotinic receptor and is blocked by curare while the receptor stimulated by muscarine is known as the muscurinic receptor and is blocked by atropine (Carlson 1998). Thus, acetylcholine produces very quick excitatory responses similar to those evoked by nicotine, and yet it also produces slow responses similar to those evoked by muscarine.

Multiple receptors exist for acetylcholine as they show subtypes (Taylor & Brown 1989). For example, nicotinic receptors found in neuromuscular junction (N_1 receptors) are different from those in ganglia (N_2 receptors). Likewise, muscarinic receptors also show distinct subtypes, namely M_1 and M_2. It is now known that M_1 receptors have a higher affinity for the drug pirenzepine (a muscarinic antagonist) while M_2 receptors have a low affinity (Taylor & Brown 1989).

Nicotinic receptors are found in peripheral ganglia and skeletal muscle. Ganglionic nicotinic receptors are found on postsynaptic neurones in both parasympathetic and sympathetic ganglia and in adrenal glands. Muscarinic receptors are the mediator of postganglionic parasympathetic neurotransmission. Some sympathetic responses such as sweating and piloerection are also mediated through muscarinic receptors. Muscarinic receptors with high affinity for pirenzepine appear to be more present in cerebral cortex, corpus striatum and hippocampus while those with low affinity for pirenzepine are mainly found in cerebellum (Taylor & Brown 1989). Muscarinic receptors are found not only in CNS and ganglia but also in visceral smooth muscle, secretory glands and endothelial cells of vasculature. Responses of these tissues to cholinergic stimulation can be excitatory or inhibitory, with the exception of endothelial cells.

Noradrenaline (norepinephrine)

Cell bodies of the neurones that produce noradrenaline are found mainly in a nucleus known as the locus coeruleus which is found in the brainstem (midbrain, pons and medulla oblongata). From the locus coeruleus, these neurones connect with the spinal cord, cerebellum, the hypothalamus and the thalamus. Indeed Barker (1991) states that noradrenaline is distributed from the locus coeruleus to the whole of the CNS.

The functions of noradrenaline are numerous. It increases alertness (Barker 1991), produces the alarm reaction or the fight-or-flight response (Atkinson et al 1993), regulates the secretion of vasopressin and oxytocin in addition to adjusting the secretion of the hypothalamic hormones that regulate the secretion of the anterior pituitary gland (Ganong 1999). Noradrenaline also produces vasoconstriction in most organs of the body by working on α_1 receptors. According to Ganong (1999) it also appears to be involved in both the control of food intake and the regulation of body temperature. The link between noradrenaline and mental illness is difficult to prove although it has been proposed by Hornykiewicz (1970 cited in Barker 1991) that noradrenaline hyperactivity is important in those who suffer from paranoid schizophrenia and that depletion of noradrenaline may lead to a depressed state (Barker 1991).

Dopamine

The cell bodies of the dopaminergic neurones are located primarily in the midbrain and can be divided into three main groups: nigrostriatal, mesocortical and tuberohypophysial. It is the nigrostriatal dopaminergic tract that degenerates in Parkinson's disease. The role of the mesocortical tract is hypothesised to be the emotional tone in schizophrenia while that of the tuberohypophysial is in the modulation of endocrine function (Berger & Barchas 1981). The main dopaminergic tract in the brain originates in substatia nigra from where axons that innervate the caudate nucleus and putamen of the corpus striatum commence. Coyle & Snyder (1981) state that nearly 80% of all the brain's dopamine is found in the corpus striatum. A diffuse but modest innervation to the forebrain is provided by dopaminergic cell bodies lying medial to the substantia nigra and the therapeutic effect of antipsychotic neuroleptic drugs has been associated with this system (Coyle & Snyder 1981).

Dopamine is the neurotransmitter in sympathetic ganglia. Several dopamine receptor subtypes are identified as D_1, D_2, D_3, D_4, and D_5 in the nervous system (Trimble 1996). Bloom et al (1985) have suggested that some dopamine neurones may be hyperactive in schizophrenia where inappropriate combinations of sensory information lead to abnormal misinterpretation of the stimulus. According to Trimble (1996), studies of the five dopamine receptors that have been isolated show that receptors 1 and 5 link with the enzyme adenylate cyclase and receptors 2, 3 and 4 link with the enzyme phospholipase c. Interestingly, phospholipase c inhibits adenylate cyclase. Other studies in humans with positron emission tomography (PET) have shown that there is a steady loss of dopamine receptors in basal ganglia with age and this loss is greater in men than in women (Trimble 1996). Dopamine modulates the control of voluntary movement and low levels result in parkinsonism. Evidence suggests that dopaminergic overactivity may be involved in the pathogenesis of schizophrenia (Trimble 1996), but this remains controversial. Elevated D_2 receptors have been shown by PET in brains of individuals suffering from schizophrenia. Dopamine appears to facilitate some pleasurable sensations and it is believed to mediate the enlivenment that individuals seek from taking amphetamines and cocaine (Bloom et al 1985).

Serotonin (5-hydroxytryptamine, 5HT)

Serotonin is an amine neurotransmitter that is found in highest concentration in blood platelets and is released by aggregating platelets (Green 1989). It is also found in the gastrointestinal tract (Gilman & Newman 1996), while lesser amounts are found in the brainstem and other parts of the brain (Hucho 1986). Thus, only about 1% of serotonin in the body is found in the CNS. In the brain, the distribution of serotonin is uneven with high concentrations being found in the hypothalamus and the brainstem, moderate concentrations in the cerebral cortex, hippocampus and striatum and low concentrations in the cerebellum (Brownstein 1981).

Within the brain the neurones of the Raphe nucleus have a high concentration of serotonin and from the Raphe nucleus axons project to the hypothalamus, thalamus and limbic system (Trimble 1996). Serotonin is formed from the amino acid tryptophan (Trimble 1996) and increased dietary intake of tryptophan can increase brain serotonin. Within the pineal gland, serotonin is converted to melatonin.

Trimble (1996) has described in detail three serotonin receptor subtypes, namely $5HT_1$, $5HT_2$ and $5HT_3$, while Gilman & Newman (1996) state that at least seven serotonin receptor subtypes are known. 5HT receptors are involved in the regulation of acetylcholine and dopamine release (Trimble 1996) and the classification is based on how information is passed.

Serotonin is involved in inducing sleep (Bloom et al 1985, Hucho 1986), in sensory perception, in temperature regulation and in control of mood and affective disorders, such as manic depressive illness (Gilman & Newman 1996).

Gamma aminobutyric acid (GABA)

The discovery of GABA in brain tissue was made independently in1950 by Eugene Roberts (Roberts & Frankel 1950) and Jorge Awapara (Awapara et al 1950). Further work by Obata & Takeda (1969) showed its release in mammalian systems, and its presence in the fourth ventricle when Purkinje cells were stimulated was demonstrated by Obata & Takeda (1969) and by Roberts et al (1984).

GABA is another ubiquitous neurotransmitter which is found in very high concentrations in many brain regions with concentrations up to 1000 times greater than those of monoamine neurotransmitters in the same regions (DeLorey & Olsen 1994). It is in highest concentrations in the substantia nigra, the globus pallidus, hippocampus, hypothalamus, cerebral cortex and within the grey matter of the spinal cord (Gilman & Newman 1996, Trimble 1996). The substantia nigra and the globus pallidus are two of the four separate units that make up the basal ganglia, a structure which has been described earlier in this chapter and whose name refers to its location at the base of the cortex (Bloom et al 1985). Many neurones that are acted upon by GABA are found in the limbic system (Bloom et al 1985).

Glucose is an efficient precursor of GABA; pyruvic acid and other amino acids also serve as precursors. The brain content of GABA is 200–1000 times greater than that of such neurotransmitters as dopamine, noradrenaline, acetylcholine and serotonin (McGeer & McGeer 1989).

The main function of GABA is to inhibit the firing of neurones (Bloom et al 1985, Costa and Guidotti 1985, McGeer & McGeer 1989, Trimble 1996). A neurone is less likely to fire as more GABA is bound to it (Bloom et al 1985). It is now well known that some anxiolytics such as benzodiazepines act by facilitating the effectiveness of GABA. The receptor for GABA has three subunits, namely α, β and γ, which differ in their sensitivity for GABA in their recognition sites for benzodiazepines.

Glycine

Glycine is a very simple amino acid in structure. It is an inhibitory neurotransmitter whose properties were first discovered by Purpura et al (1959) and by Curtis and co-workers (1961). Further work by Aprison & Werman (1965), Davidoff et al (1967), Werman et al (1968) and Logan & Snyder (1971) confirmed glycine as a neurotransmitter.

Glycine is found in the amygdala, the brainstem and within the spinal cord (McGeer & McGeer 1989, Trimble 1996). It works by opening and closing ionic channels (Trimble 1996). McGeer & McGeer (1989) report that glycine crosses the blood–brain barrier very easily and can be synthesised from glucose and other substrates, thus making it a very versatile compound in the brain. It increases chloride permeability (McGeer & McGeer 1989).

Endorphins

Endorphins (endogenous morphines) are morphine-like substances that are found in the brain (Bloom et al 1985, Trimble 1996). They include such substances as enkephalins, substance P and other opiates. Endorphins modulate pain, seem to modulate arousal and seem to play a role in modulating emotions (Bloom et al 1985). Controversial evidence for both an excess and a deficiency of endorphin activity in schizophrenia has been put forward by Watson & Heilman (1979) and Berger (1978). Others have reported catatonic-like behaviour in rats given β-endorphin that resembles the postural abnormalities seen in some schizophrenic patients

NEUROPATHOLOGY AND SCHIZOPHRENIA

Harrison (1999a) presents a comprehensive review of the literature concerning the neuropathological basis of schizophrenia. There is increasing evidence that schizophrenia may have a neurodevelopmental origin, involving a sequence of events occurring during pre- or perinatal development, resulting in failure of neural development, failure to establish synaptic connections and cytoarchictectural abnormalities (Duncan et al 1999). Attention has been focused on the neurochemical basis of schizophrenia and this focus has been on the:

- dopamininergic systems
- serotonergic systems
- glutamatergic/NMDA systems.

Overactivity of the dopaminergic system (*Dopamine hypothesis*) has been the pre-eminent theory of schizophrenia. Although some support has been obtained from findings of increased dopamine content and higher densities of D_2 receptors in schizophrenia there is still no consensus as to the nature of the supposed abnormality or evidence that dopamine has a causal role in schizophrenia (Harrison 1999a, Joyce & Meador-Woodruff 1997). Having undergone a number of revisions, the dopamine hypothesis postulates that dopaminergic overactivity in the ventral tegmental area of the midbrain results in the development of psychosis, and that hypodopaminergic activity in the frontal cortex may be the basis of the 'negative symptoms' of schizophrenia (Duncan et al 1999). There is also strong evidence to support supersensitivity of dopamine receptors (Duncan et al 1999).

The involvement of serotonin and in particular $5HT_{2A}$ receptor sites has been investigated. Lowered $5HT_{2A}$ receptor expression in the frontal cortex in schizophrenia has been reported, (Harrison 1999b). An elevated number of cortical $5HT_{1A}$ receptors is also a replicated finding (Harrison 1999a). Thus the hypotheses to explain the involvement of serotonin receptors are being refined.

Glutamatergic dysfunction has been proposed as a hypothesis for the development of schizophrenia. Mechanisms proposed to explain the involvement of glutamate focus on its interaction with dopamine (Harrison 1999a). Linked to glutamatergic dysfunction, there is evidence to implicate NMDA receptor hypofunction as well (Duncan et al 1999). NMDA antagonists activate dopaminergic neurones and hypofunction of NMDA receptors may lead to sensitisation of the dopamine system. NMDA receptor hypofunction may be the link in the pathophysiology of schizophrenia and may arise from a developmental abnormality (Duncan et al 1999).

NEUROCHEMISTRY AND AFFECTIVE DISORDERS

The classical neurochemical theory proposed was the *monoamine hypothesis* (Schildkraut & Kety 1967). In short, it was proposed that endogenous depression was caused by a functional deficit of monoamine transmitters, for example noradrenaline, while mania results from an excess. In its simplest form this hypothesis is no longer tenable and attempts have been made to revise the monoamine theory (Heninger et al 1996). Pharmacological evidence generally still supports the view that manipulation of monoaminergic systems can alleviate the symptoms of depression but the monoamine hypothesis does not explain the delay between pharmacological changes and clinical effects. Attention has moved away from neurotransmitter level and turnover to the role of pre- and postsynaptic receptors.

Dysfunction of noradrenergic and serotonergic systems still remains central to the neurochemical theories of depression (Van Praag 1980a). Cholinergic mechanisms have been implicated, with depression reflecting cholinergic dominance and mania reflecting noradrenergic excess, but the evidence is limited. Dopamine dysfunction may be involved in motor symptoms associated with depression.

Noradrenergic system

There appears to be reduced sensitivity of postsynaptic noradrenergic α receptors. Increased sensitivity of β adrenergic receptors has also been demonstrated. Indeed most, but not all, antidepressant drugs lead to downregulation (decreased activity) of postsynaptic β adrenergic receptors (Sulser 1984).

Serotonergic systems

With the introduction of selective serotonin reuptake inhibitor (SSRI) antidepressants, interest has moved to the role of serotonin receptors and in particular the interaction between pre- and postsynaptic 5HT receptors. There appears to be some evidence of abnormal function of the presynaptic $5HT_{1A}$ receptors. In addition increased sensitivity of $5HT_2$ postsynaptic receptors may be implicated.

There is some evidence to support the view that depletion of serotonin may precipiate depression and may be a trait factor linked to the susceptibility to develop depression (Van Praag 1980b). Low concentrations of serotonin uptake sites on platelets when measured by imipramine binding to platelets (Ellis & Salmon 1994) have been demonstrated in depressed patients. Low concentrations of serotonin metabolites in cerebrospinal fluid have been demonstrated in individuals who have attempted suicide (Lidberg et al 1985). This finding does not seem to be dependent on being depressed. Similar results have been observed in individuals suffering from schizophrenia who have attempted suicide but were not depressed and in patients with aggression. It may be that serotonin depletion is related to impulse control and aggression rather than depression per se (Trimble 1996).

Overall, there are still many unresolved issues regarding the neurochemical basis of affective disorders. The evidence is difficult to interpret and antidepressants themselves alter receptor function. The interaction between pre- and postsynaptic receptors is still unclear. However, changes in receptor sensitivity do go some way to explain the delayed clinical effects of antidepressants.

CONCLUSION

The role of the brain as an integration and processing centre for the vast range of information it receives should not be underestimated. The characteristic features observed in patients in terms of abnormal thought processes, lability in mood, variation in feelings and inappropriate behaviour are an output of the information that the brain receives and processes. Pathophysiological changes within both the CNS and the PNS will affect this output as can be demonstrated by the role of the thalamus, hypothalamus and basal ganglia.

Knowledge of the autonomic nervous system by mental health nurses can facilitate an understanding of whole body responses and can help nurses to work therapeutically with patients on biofeedback techniques.

The role of the limbic system and its link with various neurotransmitters support its pivotal role as a centre for regulating emotional responses to stimuli in addition to its other role as a stimuli-discriminating and storage centre. Since many drugs take effect by influencing events at the synapse, it stands to reason that it is prudent for mental health practitioners to have knowledge and understanding of the structure and function of the synapse.

Mental health nurses cannot afford to ignore the issues of cognitive impairment patterns of brain development, deranged patterns of cerebral blood flow, nutritional impact on neurological function and other neurological issues in their quest to distance themselves from biology. The real challenge according to Ron (1995) is how to integrate the various findings into a coherent whole and to link them to presumed aetiological factors. This challenge has its benefit in enabling mental health nurses to understand aspects of whole body/person responses in individuals who are mentally ill.

REFERENCES

Aprison M H, Werman R 1965 The distribution of glycine in cat spinal cord and roots. Life Sciences 4: 2075–2083

Atkinson R L, Atkinson R C, Smith E E, Bem D J 1993 Introduction to psychology, 11th edn. Harcourt Brace College Publishers, Fort Worth, Texas

Awapara J, Landau A J, Fuerst R, Seale B 1950 Free γ-aminobutyric acid in brain. Journal of Biological Chemistry 187: 35-39

Barker R A 1991 Neuroscience: an illustrated guide. Ellis Horwood, New York

Barr M L, Kiernan J A 1993 The human nervous system: an anatomical viewpoint, 6th edn. Lippincott, Philadelphia

Ben-Ari Y 1981 Transmitters and modulators in the amygdaloid complex: a review. In: Ben-Ari Y (ed) The amygdaloid complex. Elsevier, North Holland, p 163–174

Berger P A 1978 Medical treatment of mental illness. Science 200: 974–981

Berger P A, Barchas J D 1981 Biochemical hypotheses of mental disorders. In: Siegel G J, Albers R W, Agranoff B W, Katzman R (eds) Basic neurochemistry, 3rd edn. Little Brown, Boston, p 759–775

Berne R M, Levy M N 1996 Principles of physiology, 2nd edn. Mosby, St Louis, p 91–110

Bloom F E, Lazerson A, Hofstadter L 1985 Brain, mind and behaviour. W H Freeman, New York

Broca P 1878 Anatomie comparee des circonvolutions cerebrals: le grand lobe limbique et la scissure limbique dans la serie des mammiferes. In: Trimble M R 1996 Biological psychiatry, 2nd edn. Wiley, Chichester, p 76–115

Brodmann K 1909 Vergleichende lokalisationlehre der grosshirnrinde in ihren Prinzipien dargestellt auf grund des Zellenbaues, J A Barth, Leipzig

Brownstein M J 1981 Serotonin, histamine and the purines. In: Siegel G S, Albers R W, Agranoff B W, Katzman R Basic neurochemistry, 3rd edn. Little Brown, Boston, p 219–232

Cannon W B 1930 The autonomic nervous system: an interpretation. Lancet 1: Carlson N R 1998 Physiology of behaviour, 6th edn. Allyn and Bacon, Boston 1109–1115

Carlson N R 1998 Physiology of behaviour, 6th edn. Allyn and Bacon, Boston

Carpenter R H S 1996 Neurophysiology, 3rd edn. Arnold, London

Costa E, Guidotti A 1985 Endogenous ligands for benzodiazepine recognition sites. Biochemical Pharmacology 34(19): 3399–3403

Coyle J T, Snyder S H 1981 Catecholamines. In: Siegel G S, Albers R W, Agranoff B W, Katzman R (eds) Basic neurochemistry, 3rd edn. Little Brown, Boston, p 205–218

Curtis D R, Watkins J C 1960 The excitation and depression of spinal neurones by structurally related amino acids. Journal of Neurochemistry 6: 117–141

Curtis D R, Phillis J W, Watkins J C 1961 Actions of amino acids on isolated hemisected spinal cord of the toad. British Journal of Pharmacology 16: 262–283

Dale H H 1914 The action of certain esters and ethers of choline and their relation to muscarine. Journal of Pharmacology 6: 147–190

Dale H H 1935 Pharmacology and nerve endings. Proceedings of the Royal Society of Medicine 28: 319–332

Davidoff R A, Graham L T Jr, Shank R P, Werman R, Aprison M H 1967 Changes in amino acid concentrations associated with loss of spinal interneurones. Journal of Neurochemistry 14: 1025–1031

DeLorey T M, Olsen R W 1994 GABA and glycine. In: Siegel G J, Agranoff B W, Albers R W, Mohinoff P B (eds) Basic neurochemistry, 5th edn. Raven Press, New York, p 389–399

De Robertis E D P 1964 Histophysiology of synapses and neurosecretion. International series of monographs on pure and applied biology – modern trends in physiological sciences. Pergamon Press, Oxford

Duncan G E, Sheitman B B, Lieberman J A 1999 An integrated view of pathophysiological models of schizophrenia. Brain Research Reviews 29: 250–264

Ellis P M, Salmon C 1994 Is platelet imipramine binding reduced in depression? Biological Psychiatry 36: 292–300

Feldberg W, Voigt M (1948) Acetylcholine synthesis in different regions of the central nervous system. Journal of Physiology 107: 372–381

Feldberg W, Gaddum J H 1934 The chemical transmitter at synapses in a sympathetic ganglion. Journal of Physiology 81: 305

Ganong W F 1999 Review of medical physiology, 17th edn. Prentice-Hall, London.

Green P J 1989 Histamine and serotonin. In: Siegel G J, Agranoff B W, Albers R W, Molinoff P (eds) Basic neurochemistry, 4th edn. Raven Press, New York, p 253–270

Gilman S, Newman S W 1996 Manter and Gatz's essentials of clinical neuroanatomy and neurophysiology, 9th edn. F A Davis, Philadelphia

Harrison P J 1999a The neuropathology of schizophrenia: a critical review of the data and their interpretation. Brain 122: 593–624

Harrison P J 1999b Neurochemical alterations in schizophrenia affecting the putative targets of atypical antipsychotics: focus on dopamine (D_1, D_2, D_4) and $5HT_{2A}$ receptors. British Journal of Psychiatry 174 (suppl 38): 41–51

Haubrich D R, Chippendale T J 1977 Regulation of acetylcholine synthesis. Life Sciences 20: 1465–1478

Heninger G R, Delgado P L, Charney D S 1996 The revised monoamine theory of depression: a modulatory role for monamines, based on new findings from monoamine depletion experiments in humans. Pharmacopsychiatry 29: 2–11

Hille B 1992 Ionic channels of excitable membrances, 2nd edn. Sinauer Associates, Sunderland, Massachusetts

Hucho F 1986 Neurochemistry: fundamentals and concepts. VCH, Weinheim

Iversen L L 1970 Metabolism of catecholamines. In: Lajtha A 1970 (ed) Handbook of neurochemistry. Plenum Press, New York, p 197–220

Joyce J N, Meador-Woodruff J H 1997 Linking the family of D_2 receptors to neuronal circuits in human brain: insights into schizophrenia. Neuropsychopharmacology 16(6): 375–384

Kötter R, Meyer N 1992 The limbic system: a review of its empirical foundation. Behavioural Brain Research 52: 105–127

Krnjevic K 1974 Chemical nature of synaptic transmission in vertebrates. Physiology Review 54: 418–540

Lidberg L, Tuck J R, Åsberg M, Scalia-Tomba G, Betillson L 1985 Homicide, suicide and CSF 5-HIAA. Acta Psychiatrica Scandinavica 71: 230–236

Llinas R R 1988 The biology of the brain – from neurons to networks. Readings from Scientific American Magazine. W H Freeman, New York

Loewi O 1935 The Ferrier Lecture on problems connected with the principle of humoral transmission of nervous impluses. Proceedings of the Royal Society B118: 299–316

Logan W J, Snyder S H 1971 Unique high uptake systems for glycine, glutamic and aspartic acids in central nervous tissue of the rat. Nature 234: 297–299

McGeer P L, McGeer E G 1989 Amino acid neurotransmitters. In: Siegel G J, Agranoff B W, Albers R W, Molinoff P (eds) Basic neurochemistry, 4th edn. Raven Press, New York, p 311–332

MacIntosh F C 1981 Acetylcholine In: Siegel G J, Albers R W, Agranoff B W, Katzman R, Basic neurochemistry, 3rd edn. Little Brown, Boston, p 183–204

Maclean P D 1970 The triune brain, emotion and scientific bias. In: Schmidt F O, Worden F G (eds) The neurosciences, second study programme. Rockefeller University Press, New York, p 336–349

Nauta W J H, Domesick V B 1982 Neural associations of the limbic system. In: Beckman A (ed) The neural basis of behaviour. Spectrum, New York, p 175–206

Neal M J 1997 Medical pharmacology at a glance, 3rd edn. Blackwell Scientific, Oxford

Niewenhuys R 1996 The greater limbic system, the emotional motor system and the brain. In: Holstege G, Bandler R, Saper C B (eds) The emotional motor system. Elsevier, Amsterdam, p 551–580

Noback C R, Strominger N L, Demarest R J 1996 The human nervous system: structure and function, 5th edn. Williams & Wilkins, Philadelphia

Obata K, Takeda K 1969 Release of GABA into the fourth ventricle induced by stimulation of the cat cerebellum. Journal of Neurochemistry 16: 1043–1047

Papez J W 1937 A proposed mechanism of emotion. Archives of Neurology and Psychiatry 38: 725–733

Purpura D P, Girado M, Smith T G, Callan D A, Grundfest H 1959 Structure activity determinants of pharmacological effects of amino acids and related compounds on central synapses. Journal of Neurochemistry 3: 238–266

Purves D, Augustine G J, Fitzpatrick D, Katz L C, La Mantia A S, McNamara J O 1997 Neuroscience. Sinauer Associates, Sunderland, Massachusetts

Roberts E, Frankel S 1950 γ-Aminobutyric acid in brain: its formation from glutanic acid. Journal of Biological Chemistry 187: 55–63

Roberts G W, Polak J M, Crow T J 1984 Peptide circuitry of the limbic system. In: Trimble M R, Zarifian E (eds) Psychopharmacology of the limbic system. Oxford University Press, Oxford, p 226–243

Ron M 1995 Schizophrenia and the brain: where is it? MRC News: 4–5

Schildkraut J J, Kety S S 1967 Biogenic amines and emotion. Science 156: 21–30

Siegel G J, Albers R W, Agranoff B W, Katzman R 1996 Basic neurochemistry, 5th edn. Little Brown, Boston

Sulser F 1984 Regulation and function of noradrenaline receptor in systems in the brain. Neuropharmacology 23: 255–261

Taylor P, Brown J H 1989 Acetylcholine. In: Seigel G, Agranoff B, Albers R W, Molinoff P (eds) Basic neurochemistry, 4th edn. Raven Press, New York, p 203–231

Thibodeau G A, Patton K T 1993 Anatomy and physiology: international edition, 2nd edn. Mosby, St Louis

Thompson R F 1986 Progress in neuroscience. Readings from Scientific American. W H Freeman, New York

Trimble M R 1996 Biological psychiatry, 2nd edn. John Wiley, Chichester

Tucek S, Ricny J, Dolezal I V 1990 Advances in the biology of cholinergic neurones. Advances in Neurology 51: 109–115

Ulus I H, Wurtman R J, ScallyM C, Hirsch M J 1978 Effect of choline on cholinergic function. In: Jenden D J (ed) Cholinergic mechanisms and psychopharmacology. Plenum, New York, p 525–538

Van Praag H M 1980a Central monoamine metabolism in depression II. Catecholamines and related compounds. Comprehensive Psychiatry 21: 44–45

Van Praag H M 1980b Central monoamine metabolism in depression I. Serotonin and related compounds. Comprehensive Psychiatry 21: 30–43

Watson R T, Heilman K M 1979 Thalamic neglect. Neurology 29: 690–694

Werman R, Davidoff R A, Aprison M H 1968 Inhibitory effect of glycine in spinal neurones in the cat. Journal of Neurophysiology 31: 81–95.

Willis T 1664 Cerebri anatome: cui accessit nervorum descriptio et usus. Flesher, London. Cited in Brazier MABA A historical development of neurophysiology. In: Field J, Magoun H W, Hall V E (eds) 1959 Handbook of physiology, section 1: Neurophysiology, vol 1, American Physiological Society, Washington DC, p 1–58

4

Brain metabolism, hormonal activity and mental health

Key Points

- Hypoglycaemia produces behavioural and perceptual disturbances, including aggressive behaviour, disordered thought and hallucinations
- Activation of the thyroid system seems to be important in the normal response to stress and the recovery from depression
- Hypothyroidism is associated with depression
- Thyroid hormone therapy may provide benefit in refractory depression
- Hypersecretion of cortisol has been demonstrated in major depression
- The psychobiological basis of SAD remains unclear
- SAD can be reversed by light therapy
- PMS is a major distressing condition
- Abnormal serotonin secretion is also implicated in PMS

Cognitive function, behavioural responses and mood are all affected by alterations to specific metabolic and endocrine activity. The focus of this chapter is on aspects of metabolic and hormonal activity that may produce mental health problems and may affect the ability of an individual to respond to everyday factors. In particular, aspects of glucose metabolism and disorders of thyroid function are considered. Furthermore, seasonal affective disorder (SAD) and premenstrual syndrome (PMS) are discussed.

In order to function, nervous tissue, as with any other tissue such as muscle tissue, requires energy. Such energy is derived from the digestion and metabolism of nutrients. Consistent with all tissues of the body, glucose is the major nutrient from which, by a process of oxidative metabolism, energy, in the form of adenosine triphosphate, is obtained.

Metabolism refers to all the biochemical reactions that occur within an organ or within a whole organism. The brain is very active metabolically. Grey matter has a very high rate of oxidative metabolism and its oxygen consumption, which is approximately 7 ml.min^{-1}.100g^{-1}, accounts for nearly 20% of human oxygen consumption at rest (Levick 1995). Indeed, grey matter receives about 100 ml blood.min^{-1}.100 g^{-1}, which is greater than 10 times the average for the whole body, and extracts about 35% of the delivered oxygen (Levick 1995).

THE METABOLISM OF GLUCOSE

The metabolism of glucose into ATP involves three processes:

- glycolysis
- tricarboxylic acid (citric acid or Krebs) cycle
- oxidative phosphorylation.

Glycolysis occurs in the cytoplasm of all cells, including nerve cells, and accounts for approximately 5% of ATP production. Glucose is converted via several intermediary steps to pyruvate, resulting in the net production of 2-ATP. Oxygen is not utilised in this metabolic process, so glycolysis is an example of anaerobic metabolism.

The tricarboxylic cycle (citric acid or Kreb's cycle) is a series of biochemical reactions that occur in the matrix of mitochondria and is the final common pathway for the oxidation of fuel molecules. During this process the large amount of potential energy stored in the intermediate substances derived from pyruvic acid is released step by step in the form of hydrogen ions, with carbon dioxide being produced as a waste product. The liberated hydrogen ions are carried by coenzymes to the electron transport chain where oxidative phosphorylation occurs. Importantly, the tricarboxylic cycle only operates under aerobic conditions.

The electron transport chain consists of a sequence of carrier molecules located on the inner mitochondrial membrane. High energy electrons, obtained from the hydrogen ions released from the tricarboxylic acid cycle, are transferred to the carrier molecules. A series of electron transfers occur resulting in the final reaction of hydrogen atoms with oxygen to form water and ATP. This aerobic process is called oxidative phosphorylation and accounts for 95% of ATP production. The overall reaction can be summarised in a simplified form as follows:

$C_6H_{12}O_6 + 6O_2 \rightarrow 6CO_2 + 6H_2O + 36$ ATP (net)
Glucose

The availability of glucose and oxygen is crucial for the effective production of ATP and nerve cell function. As a result the autoregulation of blood flow is well developed in the brain to preserve metabolic activity.

HYPOGLYCAEMIA AND BRAIN FUNCTION

Glucose readily enters nerve cells by diffusion and, unlike muscle and fat cells, insulin is not required to facilitate the process. However, in the presence of low plasma glucose levels (hypoglycaemia) the concentration gradient between the plasma and the nerve cells is lower, resulting in less glucose entering the cells. When there is a significant deficiency in the amount of glucose in the nerve cells (glucopenia) nerve

Table 4.1   Summary of major endocrine disorders

Endocrine disorder	Significant symptoms and signs	Associated mental health problems
Hyperthyroidism	Excess thyroid hormone *Symptoms*: heat intolerance, palpitations, increased appetite with no weight gain or actual weight loss, resting tachycardia, increased sweating, insomnia, fine tremor of hands	Possible emotional lability, highly distractible, anxiety, excitability, short attention span, impaired recent memory Severe symptoms may resemble acute psychosis
Hypothyroidism	Insufficient thyroid hormone *Symptoms*: sensitive to cold, dryness of skin, coarse and dry hair, constipation, weight gain, lethargy, deafness, vague generalised aching muscles, disordered menstrual function, lowered body temperature, slow and husky speech	Depression and low mood predominant. Impaired recent memory may be present with lethargy and lack of volition Paranoid suspicions and auditory hallucinations may be present
Addison's disease	Insufficient secretion of adrenocortical hormones due to adrenal gland failure *Symptoms*: weakness, weight loss, hypotension, menstrual disorders, hyperpigmentation of the skin and vitiligo, gastrointestinal disorders including anorexia, nausea and constipation alternating with diarrhoea	Poverty of thought, apathy, fatigue, depression, psychomotor retardation Severe forms may include frank psychosis
Cushing's syndrome	Elevated corticosteroid secretion *Symptoms*: increased appetite, moon face, central obesity, hypertension, amenorrhoea, hirsutism and muscle weakness	Depression, with high risk of suicide, emotional lability, insomnia, confusion and disorientation
Hypopituitarism	Lack of pituitary hormone *Symptoms*: male – loss of libido and impotence. Female – amenorrhoea All – loss of body hair, pale skin, low body temperature, may develop coma	Apathy, indifference, depression, cognitive deficits, delusions

Adapted from Rawlins et al (1993) with permission.

cell dysfunction occurs. Symptoms of dizziness, double vision and mental confusion occur. Indeed, coupled with tremor, faintness, palpitation and sweating, one has the classical symptoms of hypoglycaemia. The degree of nerve cell dysfunction and associated mental confusion can lead to the development of inappropriate behaviour similar to that resulting from alcohol intoxication: there have been occasions when individuals have been arrested by the police for drunk and disorderly behaviour, but were then found to be hypoglycaemic.

It is imperative that mental health nurses have an understanding of the effects of changes in the levels of blood sugar and that when assessing any sudden change in the behaviour of a client, consideration is given to the possibility of the cause lying with changes in the blood sugar level.

While it is well recognised that alterations to endocrine activity can lead to mental health problems, the exact mechanisms linking hormonal activity to mood and cognitive function are not fully understood. Table 4.1 provides a brief summary of some of the major endocrine disorders that may lead to mental health disturbance. Alterations to the hypothalamic-pituitary-thyroid (HPT) axis and to the hypothalamic-pituitary-adrenal (HPA) axis have been associated with depression. Both axes rely on negative feedback mechanisms.

HYPOTHALAMIC-PITUITARY-THYROID (HPT) AXIS

The HPT axis describes the secretion of thyroid hormones. The thyroid hormones T_3 (triiodothyronine) and T_4 (thyroxine) are secreted from the thyroid gland and are involved with the regulation of cellular metabolism. The release of the thyroid hormones is influenced by thyroid stimulating hormone (TSH) secreted from the anterior pituitary gland. The secretion of TSH is itself regulated by thyrotropin-releasing hormone (TRH) secreted by the hypothalamus. The level of free T_3 and T_4 via a negative feedback mechanism influences the secretion of TSH and TRH.

The brain seems to utilise thyroid hormones differently from other tissues, with thyroid hormones having a specific uptake and discrete distribution within the brain (Dratman 1993, Haggerty & Prange 1995). Furthermore, the brain has the unique ability to control the conversion of T_4 to T_3 locally, suggesting that levels of thyroid hormone may be regulated more tightly in the brain compared to other tissues (Dratman 1993). Lastly, activation of the thyroid system seems to be an important component of the normal response to stress and the recovery from depression (Haggerty & Prange 1995).

There has been a long history in the relationship between thyroid activity and affective disorders, particularly depression. Despite methodological problems there is consistent evidence, in a subset of subjects with major depression, of a blunted response of TSH to TRH challenge and disturbances in the circadian patterns of the HPT axis (Sullivan et al 1997). Hypothyroidism has long been associated with depression and subclinical hypothyroidism has gained increasing importance. Indeed the traditional view of hypothyroidism as being present or absent has largely been superseded by the concept of a spectrum of thyroid dysfunction with different grades of subclinical hypothyroidism based on specific TSH values (Haggerty & Prange 1995, Weetman 1997). Severe hypothyroidism is associated with major depression. It also seems that the presence of subclinical hypothyroidism may be a risk factor for depression (Haggerty et al 1993). Hypothyroidism is associated with reduced central serotonin (5HT) function (Cleare et al 1996). However, it is not clear whether subclinical hypothyroidism is a primary cause of depression. The case may be that it merely compounds the effects of other stressors.

There is an increasing body of evidence that the addition of thyroid hormone therapy to existing antidepressant treatment can improve mood stabilisation in patients with bipolar affective disorder, provide benefit in the treatment of refractory depression and improve symptom scores and psychometric performance when subclinical hypothyroidism is present (Haggarty & Prange 1995, Weetman 1997). The mechanism for this is unclear but thyroxine replacement therapy has been found to increase central serotonin (5HT) activity (Cleare et al 1996). While there is conflicting evidence as to the extent of thyroid dysfunction within patients (Sullivan et al 1997), for the reasons outlined above, patients with depression should be screened for subclinical and overt hypothyroidism.

HYPOTHALAMIC-PITUITARY-ADRENAL (HPA) AXIS

The HPA axis relates to the secretion of cortisol, the principal glucocorticoid in humans. Specifically, the hypothalamus secretes corticotropin-releasing hormone (CRH) which stimulates the release of adrenocorticotropic hormone (ACTH) from the anterior pituitary gland. ACTH then stimulates the release of cortisol from the adrenal cortex. Increases in the level of plasma cortisol then via a negative feedback mechanism inhibit the secretion of CRH and therefore of ACTH. The HPA axis is responsible for the control of cortisol secretion and therefore the response to changes in the environment and adaptation to stress. Overactivity of the HPA axis results from excessive stimulation via stress and circadian rhythms and/or inadequate negative feedback control.

Overactivity of the HPA system has been demonstrated in individuals with major depression, with elevated plasma cortisol levels and 24-hour urinary free cortisol (Cooney & Dinan 1996) and with abnormal dexamethasone suppression tests (Carroll et al 1981, Trimble 1996). The dexamethasone suppression test (DST) involves suppressing the secretion

Table 4.2 Non-suppression in DST according to affective state

	Non-suppression (% of subjects)
Normal group	7.2
Acute grief	9.5
Major depressive disorder	43.1
Psychotic affective disorders (including bipolar disorders)	68.6
With suicide intent	77.8

Taken from Arana & Baldessarini (1985)

of ACTH and cortisol by administering 1–2 mg of dexamethasone (Carroll et al 1981, Silverton & Cookson 1982). While there are significant methodological issues related to interpreting the results of the DST, non-suppression has been observed in mental health conditions where depression is a feature (Carroll et al 1976). A summary of one review is given in Table 4.2. There is evidence that the abnormal DST may revert to normal following treatment and that a failure to do so is a bad prognostic sign and may signal an increased risk of suicide (Trimble 1996).

The following abnormalities in the HPA axis associated with depression have been observed (Cooney & Dinan 1996, Trimble 1996):

- overactivity of the HPA axis
- cortisol hypersecretion
- increased urinary free cortisol
- increased CSF corticotrophin-releasing factor
- increased circulating ACTH
- abnormal circadian rhythms of cortisol
- increased adrenal gland size
- altered glucocorticoid receptor sensitivity
- abnormal dexamethasone suppression test.

SEASONAL AFFECTIVE DISORDER (SAD)

The diagnosis of seasonal affective disorder (SAD) is reserved for depression that is associated with a particular time of year and season (autumn to winter) and where there is full remission during another time of year (summer). Although SAD is a diagnostic label, attention has focused on the concept of seasonality, i.e. worsening of mood and other behaviour in winter in otherwise normal individuals. Epidemiological studies have shown that there is a spectrum of seasonality in the general population with SAD representing an extreme pathological variant.

Classically SAD was described by Rosenthal et al (1984) as a syndrome characterised by recurrent episodes of depression in autumn and winter, with atypical symptoms of fatigue, increased sleep, increased anxiety, craving for carbohydrate and weight gain (Dalgleish et al 1996). In recent years variations in the age of onset of SAD have been reported. There are increasing numbers of reports of SAD in children and adolescents and also of late onset in older people (Dalgleish et al 1996). There appears to be a higher incidence in women compared to men with a female:male ratio ranging from 3.5:1 to 9.0:1 in Alaska, North America, Europe and Australia. This is in contrast to Japan where lower ratios of 1.4:1 to 1.9:1 have been reported (Okawa et al 1996).

Attention has focused on the psychobiological basis of SAD. There is strong evidence that SAD can be reversed by light exposure and a negative correlation between SAD and the total number of hours of sunshine has been demonstrated. Several theories have been proposed to explain the action of light on mood, but the psychobiological basis remains unclear. Particular attention has focused on the hormone melatonin, which is secreted from the pineal gland during darkness and is found principally in the hypothalamus and midbrain. Light inhibits the secretion of melatonin. While melatonin seems to modify the hypothalamic control of various hormones and, in animals, is important in regulating seasonal changes, alteration in melatonin secretion does not appear to be of major significance in the development of SAD (Dalgleish et al 1996). The neurotransmitters dopamine, serotonin and noradrenaline have all been implicated in the pathogenesis of SAD. Serotonin (5HT), a precursor of melatonin, may well have a prominent role in mediating seasonal affective changes. Indeed serotonin agonists can provide benefit for those with SAD, although it must be stressed that the treatment of choice remains light therapy.

LIGHT THERAPY

Much debate has centred around the most effective intensity of light, duration of exposure and time of day of exposure. There appears to be a positive correlation between the light intensity and improvement in symptoms. While some have reported that a greater effect is produced by morning exposure (Terman et al 1989), there does not appear to be a critical time of day to perform the treatment (Dalgleish et al 1996). Clinically, phototherapy involves the presentation of bright (minimum 2500 lux) artificial light, daily, for a minimum of two hours, at a time that is most convenient for the subject (Dalgleish et al 1996). It is usual for phototherapy to be administered within two weeks of the onset of symptoms and continued throughout the winter months.

Bright light does seem to produce specific antidepressant benefit over and beyond any placebo effect but it takes at least three weeks for this effect to develop (Eastman et al 1998). It seems that serotonin plays an important role in the mechanism of action of light therapy (Neumeister et al 1998). There is evidence to support that SAD is associated with aberrations in the serotonin uptake mechanism which in part may be modified by light therapy (Stain-Malmgren et al 1998). With regard to the use of antidepressant drugs, both light and fluoxetine produced similar responses, with light treatment in the morning producing a significantly faster onset of improvement (Ruhrmann et al 1998).

PREMENSTRUAL SYNDROME (PMS)

Premenstrual syndrome does not often feature in mental health textbooks, but the impact of PMS for individual women can be significant and therefore within a chapter on hormonal effects PMS needs to be included. For clarity, PMS is also called late luteal phase dysphoric disorder by the American Psychiatric Association.

PMS is a constellation of symptoms related to hormonal fluctuations occurring with the menstrual cycle. PMS is characterised by distressing physical, psychological and behavioural changes of such severity that interpersonal and other activities are adversely affected. Attempts have been made to classify milder forms of PMS and more severe but less common forms. Indeed, more recently the American Psychiatric Association has included in the appendix of the fourth edition (DSM-IV) research diagnostic criteria for a severe form of PMS called premenstrual dysphoric disorder (PMDD; American Psychiatric Association 1994). PMDD criteria emphasise that the occurrence of the symptoms must be confined to the luteal phase of the menstrual cycle. Five of 11 possible symptoms must be present, of which at least one must be depressed mood, anxiety, lability or irritability. The criteria also emphasise that social and interpersonal functioning are affected. Using such strict criteria to validate PMS establishes that not all women who have premenstrual symptoms necessarily have a mental illness. Furthermore, symptoms reported as PMS may in fact be premenstrual exacerbation of an underlying disorder not directly related to the menstrual cycle (Pearlstein 1995, Steiner 1997).

The aetiology of PMS and PMDD is still largely unknown. Female sex hormones clearly have been a central focus. However, attempts to attribute the mood changes to an excess of oestrogen, withdrawal of oestrogen, a deficit of progesterone or an imbalance in oestrogen:progesterone ratio have been inconclusive (Steiner 1997). The view that the ovarian cycle is important in the aetiology is nevertheless supported as the pharmacological suppression of ovulation results in the disappearance of premenstrual symptoms. The interactions between the normal menstrual cycle and other hormones have been investigated and other psychoneuroendocrine mechanisms triggered by the hormonal changes characteristic of the menstrual cycle have been sought.

Case study 4.1

Mary, a 35-year-old woman, was referred to a PMS clinic with severe symptoms. Her major problems were of feeling continually tired with some irritability and insomnia. Over the years a cyclical pattern to her symptoms had been identified and these had worsened during the three months prior to her visit. She also suffered from menorrhagia (heavy periods). Over the previous year she had been treated with Duphaston (dydrogesterone), a cyclical progestogen. Mary was found to have moderately severe PMS and various possible treatment options were discussed, including the use of vitamin B6 and oil of evening primrose. At this stage, oil of evening primrose was recommended and she was encouraged to complete a diary of her symptoms.

After three months, Mary reported no significant improvement following the use of evening primrose oil. She was now experiencing migraine episodes linked to her menstrual cycle. She was commenced on danazol daily in order to control her heavy periods as well as the PMS. Prozac (fluoxetine) was suggested, but at this stage Mary was reluctant to commence it. After a further three months the symptoms of heavy bleeding had stopped but the PMS continued. Approximately 15 months after the initial consultation, following minimal success from previous strategies, Prostap (leuprorelin acetate: a gonadorelin analogue) was commenced to stop the menstrual cycle. Apart from producing hot flushes this treatment was successful in abolishing the cyclicity. Hormone replacement therapy (HRT) was also introduced.

After 3.5 years following the initial consultation Mary continues on the low-dose oestrogen (20 µg) combined pill. Prozac had also been commenced and at present her mood changes have improved considerably.

Comment

This case exemplifies the difficulty in assisting women with severe PMS. There are no short-term solutions and any treatment is long term. Gonadorelin analogues with HRT help to confine the cyclical nature of the syndrome and offer a limited successful break in the remorseless continuity of the matter. Antidepressants do have a place in correcting the mood swings.

So far, investigations into the central neurotransmitter serotonin (5HT) have proved most hopeful. The serotonergic system seems to have a close reciprocal relationship with gonadal hormones, particularly androgens, and a reduction in peripheral platelet serotonin levels has been demonstrated in women with PMS (Steiner 1997). Evidence seems to be accumulating that abnormal synthesis or release of brain serotonin in the raphe nucleus, located in the brainstem, is involved in the pathogenesis of PMDD, particularly where carbohydrate craving is a feature.

Therapeutic approaches to aiding women with premenstrual disorders range from conservative lifestyle changes to treatment with hormonal therapy and antidepressants, or even surgical intervention in extreme cases. A plethora of information is available in women's journals on lifestyle changes and stress management. Furthermore the National Association for Premenstrual Syndrome (NAPS) has various publications available for advice. Attention has been given to the possible benefit dietary changes: carbohydrate consumption without protein has been shown to improve mood levels by increasing the uptake of tryptophan into the brain, resulting in increased serotonin synthesis and release (Spring & Chiodo 1987). Indeed the NAPS recommends regular intake of complex carbohydrate throughout the waking day and throughout the menstrual cycle to prevent low blood sugar levels. Homoeopathic remedies have been popularised and some efficacy has been reported in the use of vitamin B6 (pyridoxine) and evening primrose oil. However, no homoeopathic drug has been shown to be effective in multicentred randomised controlled trials and in a recent systematic review, due to the low quality of most of the trials, conclusions are limited, although the reviewers suggest that vitamin B6 up to 100 mg per day may be of benefit (Wyatt et al 1999).

For women with severe PMS and PMDD, treatment may involve manipulation of the menstrual cycle using oral contraceptives or hormonal implants. Antidepressant therapy also may be indicated. Selective serotonin reuptake inhibitors (SSRIs), such as fluoxetine and paroxetine, which modify the level of brain serotonin, have been shown to be beneficial.

DEPRESSION AND THE MENOPAUSE

There is no doubt that the menopause is a time of significant changes in a woman's life. Hunter (1996) states that besides oestrogen and progesterone levels being reduced at certain points of the menstrual cycle, both hormones are also decreased after childbirth and after the menopause. Observations have shown that during pregnancy when progesterone levels are high, some psychiatric conditions do improve thus suggesting that there is a relationship between levels of sex steroids and psychiatric morbidity. However, Hunter (1996) argues that it is rather simplistic to attribute depression to changes in hormonal levels since a complex interaction exists between several factors that include predisposing, precipitating, physical, psychological and social factors. Pugh et al (1963) and Silverton & Cookson (1982) offer the explanation that since oestrogens resemble antipsychotic drugs in their ability to oppose the effects of dopamine, pregnancy protects the expectant mother against a psychotic illness during the period of gestation.

CONCLUSION

Mental health professionals cannot dismiss the effects of the endocrine system and cellular metabolism on cognitive, behavioural and affective function. This chapter has provided an overview of the effects of endocrine and metabolic dysfunction on mental health.

REFERENCES

American Psychiatric Association 1994 Diagnostic and statistical manual for mental disorders, 4th edn. American Psychiatric Association, Washington DC

Arana G W, Baldessarini R J 1985 The dexamethasone suppression test for diagnosis and prognosis in psychiatry. Archives of General Psychiatry 42: 1193–1204

Carroll B J, Curtis G C, Mendels J 1976 Neuroendocrine regulation in depression. I. Limbic system-adrenocortical dysfunction. Archives of General Psychiatry 33: 1039–1044

Carroll B J, Feinberg M, Greden J F, Tarika J, Albaba A A, Hasket R F 1981 A specific laboratory test for the diagnosis of melancholia. Archives of General Psychiatry 38: 15–23

Cleare A J, McGregor A, Chambers S M, Dawling S, O'Keane V 1996 Thyroxine replacement increases central 5–hydroxytryptamine activity and reduces depressive symptoms in hypothyroidism. Neuroendocrinology 64: 65–69

Cooney J M, Dinan T G 1996 Preservation of hypothalamic-pituitary-adrenal axis fast-feedback responses in depression. Acta Psychiatrica Scandinavica 94: 449–453

Dalgleish T, Rosen K, Marks M 1996 Rhythm and blues: the theory and treatment of seasonal affective disorder. British Journal of Clinical Psychology 35: 163–182

Dratman M B 1993 Cerebral versus peripheral regulation and utilization of thyroid hormones. In: Joffee R J, Levitt A J (eds) The thyroid axis and psychiatric illness. American Psychiatric Association Press, New York

Eastman C I, Young M A, Fogg L F, Liu L, Meaden P M 1998 Bright light treatment of winter depression: a placebo controlled trial. Archives of General Psychiatry 55: 883–889

Haggerty J J, Prange A J 1995 Borderline hypothyroidism and depression. Annual Review of Medicine 46: 37–46

Haggerty J J, Stern R A, Mason G A, Beckwith J, Morey C E, Prange A J 1993 Subclinical hypothyroidism: a modifiable risk factor for depression? American Journal of Psychiatry 150: 508–510

Hunter M S 1996 Depression and the menopause (editorial). British Medical Journal 313:1217–1218

Levick J R 1995 An introduction to cardiovasular physiology, 2nd edn. Butterworths, London

Neumeister A, Turner E H, Mathews J R et al 1998 Effects of tryptophan depletion versus catecholamine depletion in patients with seasonal affective disorder in remission with light therapy. Archives of General Psychiatry 55: 524–530

Okawa M, Shirakawa S, Uchiyama M et al 1996 Seasonal variation of mood and behaviour in a healthy middle-aged population in Japan. Acta Psychiatrica Scandinavica 94: 211–216

Pearlstein T B 1995 Hormones and depression: what are the facts about premenstrual syndrome, menopause, and hormone replacement therapy? American Journal of Obstetrics and Gynecology 173: 646–653

Pugh T F, Jerath B K, Schmidt W M, Reed R M 1963 Rates of mental disease relating to childbearing. New England Journal of Medicine 268: 1224–1228

Rawlins R P, Williams S R, Beck C K 1993 Mental health-psychiatric nursing: a holistic life-cycle approach. Mosby Year Book, St Louis

Rosenthal N E, Sack D A, Gillin J C et al 1984 Seasonal affective disorder: a description of the syndrome and preliminary findings with light treatment. Archives of General Psychiatry 41: 72–80

Ruhrmam S, Kasper S, Hawellek B, Martinez B, Hoflich G, Nickelsen T, Moller H J 1998 Effects of fluoxetine versus bright light in the treatment of seasonal affective disorder. Psychological Medicine 28: 923–933

Silverton T M, Cookson J 1982 The biology of mania. In: K Granville-Grossman (ed) Recent advances in clinical psychiatry. Churchill Livingstone, Edinburgh, p 201

Spring B, Chiodo D J 1987 Carbohydrates, tryptophan and behaviour: a methodological review. Psychiatric Bulletin 102: 234–256

Stain-Malmgren R, Kjellman B F, Aberg-Wistedt A 1998 Platelet serotonergic functions and light therapy in seasonal affective disorder. Psychiatry Research 78: 163–172

Steiner M 1997 Premenstrual syndromes. Annual Review of Medicine 48: 447–455

Sullivan P F, Wilson D A, Mulder R T, Joyce P R 1997 The hypothalamic-pituitary-thyroid axis in major depression. Acta Psychiatrica Scandinavica 95: 370–378

Terman M, Terman J S, Quitkin F M, McGrath P J 1989 Light therapy for seasonal affective disorder: a review of efficacy. Neuropsychopharmacology 2: 1–22

Trimble M R 1996 Biological psychiatry, 2nd edn. Wiley, Chichester

Weetman A P 1997 Hypothyroidism: screening and subclinical disease. British Medical Journal 314: 1175–1178

Wyatt K M, Dimmock P W, Jones P W, Shaughn O'Brien P M 1999 Efficacy of vitamin B6 in the treatment of premenstrual syndrome: systematic review. British Medical Journal 318: 1375–1381

5

Genetic aspects

Key Points

- Inheritance deals with the passage of hereditary traits or characteristics from one generation to another
- There are 23 pairs of chromosomes in the human cell
- The genetic basis of some mental health conditions can be seen in family studies, twin studies and adoption studies
- Concordance rates in monozygotic and dizygotic twins suggest the genetic contribution in some conditions or illnesses
- It is unlikely that a single gene exists as a major risk factor for mental illnesses
- Many non-specific minor genes, and not single genes, may act together to produce a predisposition to illness
- The risk of developing a mental illness is higher where both parents are affected
- Both genes and the environment are important in many mental illnesses and dimensions of normal behaviour

This chapter deals with issues relating inheritance to mental health and mental illness. Some definitions of common genetic terminologies are given and modes of inheritance are described and discussed. The interaction of genes with non-genetic factors and linkage strategies are considered, and concordance ('agreement') rates in monozygotic and dizygotic twins are compared with the general population.

Inheritance deals with the passage of hereditary characteristics or traits from one generation to another. Genetics is the branch of biology that deals with the inheritance of traits. Before the issues relating to genetics and mental health are explored, it is necessary to explain a few terminologies.

GENETIC TERMINOLOGY

The nucleus of each human cell, excluding the gametes, contains 23 pairs (diploid number) of chromosomes. One pair is classified as sex chromosomes (X and Y) and the remaining 22 pairs as autosomes. Sex chromosomes are involved with the determination of gender, while autosomes determine the expression of other characteristics. Chromosomes arrange themselves into homologous pairs, i.e. the chromosomes that form the pair contain similar but not identical genes. Genes that determine the same characteristic, such as eye colour or height, and are located on the same position on each homologous chromosome are called alleles or allelic genes. Allelic genes may be identical and control a single characteristic. In this situation the person is said to be homozygous for the particular characteristic. When the allelic genes are different, the person is said to be heterozygous for the characteristic. The term *linkage* is used to describe genes or DNA sequences that are situated close together on the same chromosome and tend to segregate together, and *concordance* refers to the presence of the same trait in both members of a pair of twins (Kingston 1989). Genotype and phenotype are two other terms used in genetics. Genotype refers to the genetic make-up of an individual, and phenotype refers to how the genetic make-up is expressed in the body or appearance of an individual.

Sometimes one gene may suppress the expression of the other allelic gene. In this case the gene is described as being dominant. The gene that is suppressed is said to be a recessive gene. Dominant genes are expressed in the phenotype when they are present in the homozygous or heterozygous state. Recessive genes are expressed only when there are two copies present on the allele, i.e. in the homozygous state. If only one copy of the recessive gene is present, the characteristic determined by that recessive gene is not expressed and the individual can be described as being a carrier for that particular characteristic. Therefore, specific types of inheritance can be described as recessive or dominant. Indeed inheritance may be described as sex-linked if the particular inherited characteristic is located on the X or Y chromosome.

Finally, each individual inherits a unique genotype. Apart from the random fertilisation of the ova by spermatozoa, another reason for this is that during the development of ova and spermatozoa, a crossing over and exchange of regions of chromosomes takes place. The question to be asked is: is there a genetic basis for mental health problems? It has been shown that the biological children of depressed parents are more likely to experience depression than children of non-depressed parents, even when the children are raised by different parents from their biological ones (Holmes 1991). Indeed it has been known for centuries that alcohol dependence tends to run in families, and while this may not be viewed as politically correct today, Aristotle wrote 'Drunken women bring forth children like themselves' and Plato, his teacher, stated 'One drunkard begets another' (Rose 1994).

Carson et al (2000) remind us that direct visual examination of chromosomes coupled with biochemical analysis of genetic material and enzymatic processes have added to previous studies that focused on incidence of abnormalities in generations of families and on pedigree descriptions. It is generally accepted that the genetic contribution to different diseases varies, with some disorders being due entirely to environmental factors and others to genetic factors. Kingston (1989) states that many disorders do not follow simple patterns of inheritance within a family and such disorders have what is described as multifactorial or polygenic inheritance. Thus, in behavioural disorders, there is a general feeling by geneticists that the disorders do not follow Mendelian laws of inheritance but are due to a combination of many genes acting together to produce a behavioural trait or characteristic. However, it must be acknowledged that finding genetic causes is not easy due to the interaction of environmental factors with the genetic potential (Murray & Huelskoetter 1991).

In mental illness, both predisposing and precipitating factors are important. Murray & Huelskoetter (1991) define predisposing factors as those that render the person susceptible or vulnerable and are present over a period of time, while precipitating factors are events that precede the onset of the disorder or illness and occur intermittently throughout the lifetime of the individual. This means that an individual's vulnerability to precipitating factors is determined by predisposing factors. Therefore it is logical to deduce that while the exact actual behaviour expressed by an individual may depend on various prenatal, postnatal, parenting and sociological factors, genes do determine the foundation for predisposition. Family studies, twin studies and studies of adoptees do support the genetic basis for some mental health conditions.

FAMILY STUDIES

In family studies a comparison of the incidence of an illness is made between the relatives of probands (individuals with the condition under study) and the relatives of non-affected controls (Hope 1994). Since members of the general population are used for controls, Hope (1994) states that matching subjects under study for age and sex is important.

ADOPTION STUDIES

Adoption studies offer the opportunity to study individuals who have been separated from their biological parents early in life and are brought up by unrelated people, thus providing an unambiguous separation of genetic (nature) and environmental (nurture) influences for specific traits (Kendell & Zealley 1993). Both the adoptees and their families are studied and the rate of illness in adoptees versus controls as in biological parents versus adoptive parents are examined.

TWIN STUDIES

In twin studies the prevalence of the condition or disease in monozygotic twins is compared with that in dizygotic twins. Monozygotic twins are derived from a single fertilised egg and have identical genotypes whereas the genetic similarity between dizygotic twins, who are produced by the separate fertilisation of two different eggs, is about 50% (Carlson 1998).

SCHIZOPHRENIA

Luxenburger (1928 cited in Holmes 1991) was the first to report a systematic study of schizophrenia among twins. Since then several studies have compared concordance rates for schizophrenia between monozygotic and dizygotic twins. The results of these studies show a higher concordance rate of schizophrenia among monozygotic than among dizygotic twins (Fig. 5.1) and have been summarised by Holmes (1991). Other studies by Rosenthal (1961) have shown that some correlation exists between the twins in the degree to which they are disturbed. This is supported by Gottesman & Shields (1972) and by Kringlen (1967). Thus there is enough evidence to support the fact that the risk for schizophrenia is higher for individuals with relatives who suffer from schizophrenia.

According to Zerbin-Rudin (1972), children whose parents have both suffered from schizophrenia have a risk of between 40% and 68%, and those with one parent who had suffered with schizophrenia have a risk of between 9% and 16%. When a non-twin sibling has schizophrenia, the risk is reduced slightly to between 8% and 14%. Step-siblings and half-siblings of an individual with schizophrenia have a risk of 1–8% and 1–7% respectively. Grandchildren show a risk of 2–8%, cousins 2–6% and nieces and nephews 1–4% (Zerbin-Rudin 1972). The general population has a risk of 1%.

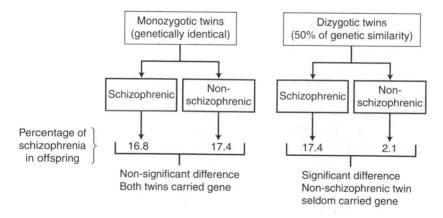

Figure 5.1 An explanation for evidence that people can have an unexpressed schizophrenia gene. Adapted from Carlson (1998).

Reviews of more recent family and twin studies by Kringlen (1990) suggest that children whose mothers have schizophrenia have an 11% chance and those whose fathers have schizophrenia have a 5% chance of suffering from schizophrenia even though the genetic correlation is the same ($r = 0.50$). This may suggest that the psychosocial influence of the mother upon her children is more important than that of the father although this suggestion may be viewed as controversial. Other studies by Goldstein et al (1990, 1992) have demonstrated that relatives of female probands are at a higher risk for schizophrenia than those of male probands.

Different chromosomes have been suggested by different groups at different times for the location of the schizophrenia gene. One possible location for the schizophrenia gene is the long arm on chromosome 5 (Bassett et al 1988) and this location and view have been confirmed and supported by other studies using DNA markers (Sherrington et al 1988). However, other workers (Crow et al 1989) have suggested that the X chromosome is involved, and have proposed that exchange of genetic material, a process known as crossing over, occurs between the short arms of the X and Y chromosomes during spermatogenesis (sperm production).

Carlson (1998) states that the exact location of the gene causing schizophrenia after crossing over can either be on the Y chromosome or remain on the X chromosome. A pseudoautosomal segment is formed after crossing over because the genes act as if they were on an autosome. Thus, according to Carlson (1998), a father will give schizophrenia to his daughters if the gene that causes schizophrenia ends up on the X chromosome, and to his sons if it ends up on the Y chromosome. Studies by Crow et al (1989) and Gorwood et al (1992) have confirmed that when more than one sibling has schizophrenia, the affected children are more than likely to be of the same sex when the history of schizophrenia is on the father's side than if it is on the mother's side. From this observation, Crow et al (1989) deduced that this difference was due to the fact that the gene for schizophrenia is located on the pseudoautosomal region.

Wei et al (1993) argue that while it is not clear whether physiological factors or genetic factors contribute more to the gender differences that are seen in schizophrenia, there is no doubt that the possibility of the link between genetic factors and gender differences in schizophrenia is a real one. Hafner et al (1989) have shown that the age of onset is earlier in schizophrenic men than in schizophrenic women while Goldstein & Link (1988) have demonstrated that male patients are generally more severely ill than are female patients. Other workers (Gittelman-Klein & Klein 1969, Goldstein 1988, Salokangas 1983, Seeman 1986) have shown that men have a poorer premorbid picture and a poorer outcome than women.

> **Case study 5.1**
>
> Pat is a 34-year-old woman who suffers from a schizophrenic illness and has been ill for the past five years. She was previously married and has a 14-year-old son and has previously lived with her son and her elderly mother. Over the past two years, however, she has become a serious risk to her elderly mother as she has attacked her on several occasions and is now living in a mental health hostel restrained by a guardianship order. She hears the voices of several men including her father who are usually criticising and berating her. At times her father tells her to kill her mother. She is taking large doses of major tranquillisers and frequently self-harms.
>
> Her father died approximately 10 years ago and himself suffered from a chronic or enduring schizophrenic illness and had numerous admissions to hospital. He was a violent man and sexually abused two of his daughters including Pat. Pat has frequent flashbacks of the abuse. She has three other sisters: two are professionals who work full-time and are married; the other sister is two years older than Pat, also suffers from schizophrenia and is in a long-stay mental health hospital in a neighbouring city. Recently one of the two professional sisters has visited her and has reported sadly that she herself has become just like her father, in that she is apathetic and withdrawn and shows very little affective warmth.

ALCOHOLISM

While the prevalence of alcoholism in the general population is 3–5% in males and 0.1% in females, it is known that 25% of close male relatives and 5–10% of close female relatives of alcoholics are themselves alcoholics (Rose 1994). The same author reports that adoption studies have found that sons of alcoholics are almost four times more likely to become alcoholic themselves than the sons of non-alcoholics, irrespective of whether their alcoholic biological parents or their non-alcoholic foster parents brought them up. Earlier studies by Goodwin et al (1973) have indicated a small genetic predisposition for alcohol abuse as shown by the fact that adopted children raised apart from their alcoholic parents show an increased incidence of alcohol abuse.

Further studies by McClearn & Hofer (1997) on gender differences in heritability of alcohol use in octogenarian (aged 80–90 years) and non-octogenarian twins found that heritability of alcohol use decreases with age and is higher in females than in males. The same authors found intra-class correlations for female monozygotic twins of 0.58 and dizygotic twins of 0.35, while for males the correlations for monozygotic and dizygotic twins were 0.08 and 0.11 respectively. They estimate that the maximum likelihood of shared heritability and unique environmental influences showed that alcohol use in females was substantially heritable at 65% with no significant shared environmental influences. On the other hand, there were no significant genetic or shared environmental influences found in males.

Table 5.1 Correlation for alcohol dependence

Twin pair	Correlation for alcohol dependence
Monozygotic female	0.54
Monozygotic male	0.47
Dizygotic female	0.36
Dizygotic male	0.24
Dizygotic male–female	0.16

Other studies over a three-year period by Kendler & Prescott (1997) (Table 5.1) on more than 6700 adult twins, which concentrated on the number of dependence symptoms and amount consumed during period of heaviest consumption, supported some of the findings by McClearn & Hofer (1997) that a substantial proportion of the risk for alcohol abuse was inherited. Kendler & Prescott (1997) conclude from the preliminary evidence that men and women share some but not all of the genetic and environmental risk factors for alcohol-related problems and behaviours.

Similar Australian surveys by Madden et al (1997) on the familial association between lifetime smoking and alcohol dependence using 2000 adult Australian twin pairs by questionnaire and telephone interviews found substantial genetic influences specific to alcohol tolerance of 50% in women and 23% in men. For smoking initiation, the figures were 81% in women and 71% in men.

Rose et al (1997) report the results of both genetic and familial–environmental influences on individual differences in the use/abuse of alcohol during adolescence in 853 Finnish twins aged 18.5 years. All twins were living with both parents. They found that the correlations for male–female twin pairs were much lower than those for female or male pairs, thus suggesting significant sex limitation of either shared genes or environmental effects. All twin correlations for consumption were found to be higher in rural than in urban environments. They concluded that in late adolescence, twin correlations for use/abuse of alcohol were modulated by urbanisation and unemployment that were characteristic of the environments in which the twins lived. Further studies by Xian et al (1997) investigated the genetic and non-genetic contributions to the association between nicotine and alcohol dependence in monozygotic and dizygotic male–male twin pairs of the Vietnam Era Twin Registry. Their findings reveal that familial factors influencing nicotine and alcohol dependence were solely due to genetic contributions comprising of 60% and 55% of total variances of nicotine and alcohol dependence respectively. They report a high genetic correlation between nicotine dependence and alcohol dependence of 0.68, with 46% of the genetic contribution to alcohol dependence being shared with the genetic contribution to nicotine dependence. This supports the view that a common genetic source for nicotine and alcohol dependence exists, even though this may be partial.

ANXIETY DISORDERS

There is evidence to support that generalised anxiety disorders, phobias and panic attacks may be inherited. There is certainly a familial pattern evident, particularly in women (Kendler et al 1992). Torgensen (1983) demonstrated a link between panic disorders and inheritance. Monozygotic twins are five times more likely to develop panic attacks than dizygotic twins.

An interesting summary of the possible link between genetic and pathophysiological anxiety is given by Murray & McGuffin (1993). They cite the parent and sibling studies of Noyes et al (1978) who, using structured interviews, showed that the risk for female relatives was twice that for male relatives. The risk for anxiety disorder when neither parent was affected was 9% but this risk rose to 24% where one parent was affected and to 44% where both parents were affected. Work by Cloninger et al (1981) found an 8% prevalence of anxiety disorder in relatives of affected individuals but only a 3% prevalence in relatives of controls. Other studies in the USA have suggested that panic disorder is familial while generalised anxiety is not (Crowe et al 1980, Noyes et al 1978).

AFFECTIVE DISORDER

Although most investigators agree that affective disorder exists in some families, it is difficult to estimate the lifetime expectancy of the disorder in the different classes of relatives (Murray & McGuffin 1993). The same authors state that a re-examination and reanalysis of previous unipolar and bipolar twin studies suggest that bipolar disorder is more genetic than unipolar disorder. In their Danish studies with 110 same-sex pairs in which at least one twin had suffered from affective disorder, Bertelsen et al (1977) showed concordance rates of 54% for unipolar and 79% for bipolar affective illness in monozygotic twins and 24% for unipolar and 19% for bipolar in dizygotic twins. Thus these studies suggest the strong genetic contribution to affective illness and that the monozygotic: dizygotic concordance ratio is higher in bipolar than in unipolar disorder (Murray & McGuffin 1993). In another British study, McGuffin et al (1991) confirm that there is a significant and substantial genetic contribution to major depression with a concordance rate of 53% in monozygotic twins compared with 28% in dizygotic twins.

Since some evidence suggests that suicidal ideation has a genetic component exerting its action on behaviour, possibly through serotoninergic neuronal pathways and also on thought content, Dikeos et al (1997) examined familial aggregation of suicidal thoughts of 28 Greek patients (13 males and 15 females) with a history of major depression belonging to 10 multi-affected families. They paired each of the 28 patients with every other patient in his or her family, resulting in 58 intrafamily pairs. Further matching for diagnosis and sociodemographic characteristics resulted in 58 interfamily pairs. Their studies found that 50 of the 58 intrafamily pairs were concordant for the presence or absence of serious suicidal thoughts while 39 of the 58 interfamily pairs showed a similar concordance with the intra/interfamily difference being more pronounced for males than for females. They concluded that familial factors play a role in the emergence of suicidal thoughts, particularly in males.

Other family studies by Jain et al (1997) compared first-degree relatives of 50 individuals who developed bipolar disorder in adolescence (mean age at onset 16.6 years) with 36 individuals who developed it as adults (mean age at onset 34.1 years). They found that the relatives of probands with a young age at onset were at greater risk of developing affective disorder. Lifetime risks were for both major depression and bipolar disorder in relatives of younger probands and the risks were independent of the gender of the proband and the relative. They also found that female relatives in both groups were more frequently affected and showed an excess of major depression with a ratio of 2:1 while bipolar disorder and major depression were equally common in male relatives with a ratio of 1:1. Their results confirm that the development of major depression at a very young age seems to have a significant genetic influence.

Early results of the variation in suicide risk in 770 relatives among 79 bipolar families reported by Simpson et al (1997) show that the risk of attempting suicide was higher among relatives of the 30 probands who had attempted suicide, occurring in 23% of their relatives versus 13% of relatives of probands with no reported attempts. Some linkage of bipolar disorder to markers on chromosome 18 was found in 28 families. There is also some suggestion that paternal transmission of bipolar disorder may be associated with a high risk of suicide.

Studies by Lenzinger et al (1997) to ascertain whether the alleles and genotypes of various serotonin receptor genes and the serotonin transporter are associated with seasonal affective disorder (SAD) indicated the possibility that the $5HT_{2A}$ receptor gene may be involved in the occurrence of SAD, thus supporting the hypothesis that serotonin is important in the pathobiology of SAD.

Case study 5.2

Phyllis is a 58-year-old woman who is married and has a grown-up son. She has a long history of a bipolar affective disorder, having both depressive and hypermanic mood swings that led to frequent admissions to hospital. She also has a degenerative eye condition and is now only partially sighted. She is a very intelligent woman who continues to teach English on a one-to-one basis with local children. Over the years she has had considerable marital problems but remains in her marriage. She is a regular attender at the local Manic Depressive Fellowship meetings and is a good organiser. She has been taking lithium for many years and when she has previously stopped this medication she has become unwell and required hospital admission. When she is hypermanic she also becomes quite paranoid, feels that people are talking about her and is frightened of persecution.

Phyllis has an identical twin sister with whom she grew up in the same family but Phyllis left home at the age of 18 years while her twin sister stayed at home. In discussion with the twin sister's consultant psychiatrist, it becomes clear that Phyllis's sister has a very similar illness and also has had regular admissions to hospital from an even younger age than Phyllis. Her marriage broke up some years previously and because of this she had less support and structure to her life and also began to drink heavily. When she becomes hypermanic, she also becomes paranoid and fearful of persecution and displays many of the other features of her sister's mental state when she is depressed. She also has been on lithium medication for a number of years and, although she has been tried on other mood stabilisers, it has been found that lithium has been the most effective drug for her, although she has still required admissions at times even when taking this medication.

Phyllis's father suffered from recurrent bouts of depression throughout his life but there is no other known history of mental illness in the family.

CONCLUSION

Due to the nature of mental illness, the genetic basis of the various mental health conditions is not that straightforward. A summary of the findings that have been discussed in this chapter is given in Table 5.2. Details and references underpinning the summary can be found in the text. Although Szasz (1976) rejects all the theories that have been advanced for the causation of schizophrenia, whether they be biochemical, genetic, familial or psychodynamic, and considers the development of modern psychiatry as the greatest scientific scandal of the scientific age, there is no doubt that the heterogeneity of schizophrenia seems to have been recognised (Tsuang et al 1990, 1991). While Owen & McGuffin (1992) favour the oligogenic hypothesis that two or three genes may be responsible for schizophrenia, Portin & Alanen (1997) argue and support the view that in the case for schizophrenia, it is unlikely that a single gene exists as a major risk factor but that many non-specific minor genes act together and lead to a predisposition to schizophrenia. The same authors advocate an integrative approach to the study of schizophrenia encompassing biopsychiatric, genetic, psychological and social-psychological perspectives. This is further

Table 5.2 Genetic findings in mental health

Condition	Summary of findings
Schizophrenia	Higher concordance among monozygotic compared to dizygotic twins Strong correlation between monozygotic twins and degree of mental health disturbance compared to dizygotic twins Stronger risk of developing schizophrenia when both parents also have schizophrenia compared to when only one parent has schizophrenia Some evidence to suggest that children are more at risk of developing schizophrenia if the mother rather than the father has schizophrenia Abnormal gene may be on chromosome 5 or the X chromosome: a pseudoautosomal segment may be formed after crossing over during meiosis
Alcoholism	Alcohol abuse seems to have a genetic basis In older people heritability is stronger in females than in males There is a view that a common genetic source exists for nicotine and alcohol dependence
Anxiety disorder	A link exists between panic disorder and inheritance The risk for developing anxiety disorder is greater when both parents have anxiety disorder compared to one parent
Affective disorder	Bipolar disorders have a stronger genetic link than unipolar disorders Concordance is greater for monozygotic twins than for dizygotic twins Heritability seems to be linked to the age of onset of the condition in the parent There is some evidence to suggest that chromosome 8 may be involved

supported by Owen & McGuffin (1997) who argue that there is little prospect of geneticists identifying the gene for schizophrenia, bipolar depression or anxiety aggression but that a consensus has begun to emerge that both genes and the environment are important in many mental illnesses and dimensions of normal behaviour. Indeed this same approach that encompasses different facets and perspectives can be advocated for other mental health conditions and it is our view that the issues raised in this chapter about genetic contribution to mental illness should be considered not in a reductionist approach but as a holistic picture.

REFERENCES

Bassett A, McGillivray B C, Jones B D, Pantzar J 1988 Partial trisomy chromosome 5 co-segregating with schizophrenia. Lancet I: 799–801
Bertelsen A, Harrald B, Hange M 1977 A Danish twin study of manic depressive disorders. British Journal of Psychiatry 130: 330–351

Carlson N R 1998 Physiology of behaviour, 6th edn. Allyn & Bacon, Boston

Carson R C, Butcher J N, Mineka S 2000 Abnormal psychology and modern life, 11th edn. Allyn & Bacon, Boston

Cloninger C R, Martin R L, Clayton P et al 1981 A blind follow up and family study of anxiety neurosis. In: Klein D F, Rabkin J (eds) Anxiety: new research and changing concepts. Raven Press, New York

Crow T J, Delisi L E, Johnstone E C 1989 Concordance by sex in sibling pairs with schizophrenia is paternally inherited. British Journal of Psychiatry 155: 92–97

Crowe R R, Pauls D A, Slymen D J, Noyes R 1980 A family study of anxiety neurosis. Archives of General Psychiatry 37: 77–79

Dikeos D G, Papadimitriou G N, Soldatos C R, Stefanis C N 1997 Suicidal thoughts in patients with major depression: a family study. American Journal of Medical Genetics, 74(6): 588

Gittelman-Klein R, Klein D 1969 Premorbid asocial adjustment and prognosis in schizophrenia. Journal of Psychiatric Research 7: 35–53

Goldstein J M 1988 Gender differences in the course of schizophrenia. American Journal of Psychiatry 145: 684–689

Goldstein J M, Link B G 1988 Gender and expression of schizophrenia. Journal of Psychiatric Research 22: 141–155

Goldstein J M, Faraone S V, Chen W J, Tolomiczencko G S, Tsuang 1990 Sex differences in familial transmission of schizophrenia. British Journal of Psychiatry 156: 819–826

Goldstein J M, Faraone S V, Chen W J, Tsuang M T 1992 Gender and familial risk for schizophrenia: disentangling confounding factors. Schizophrenia Research 7: 135–140

Goodwin D, Schulsinger F, Hermansen 1973 Alcohol problems in adoptees raised apart from alcoholic biological parents. Archives of General Psychiatry 28: 243–289

Gorwood P, Leboyer M, D'Amato T et al 1992 Evidence for a pseudoautosomal locus for schizophrenia I. A replication study using phenotype analysis. British Journal of Psychiatry 161: 55–58

Gottesman I, Shields J 1972 Schizophrenia and genetics: a twin study vantage point. Academic Press, New York

Hafner H, Riecher A, Maurer K, Loffler W, Munk-Jorgensen P, Stromgren E 1989 How does gender influence age at first hospitalization for schizophrenia? A transnational case register study. Psychological Medicine 19: 903–918

Holmes D 1991 Abnormal psychology. Harper Collins, New York

Hope R A 1994 Causes of mental illness. In: Rose N D B (ed) Essential psychiatry, 2nd edn. Blackwell Scientific, London, p 17

Jain S, Somanath C P, Reddy Y C J, Subbukrishna D K 1997 A comparative family genetic study of early and late onset bipolar disorder. American Journal of Medical Genetics (Neuropsychiatric Genetics) 74(6): 592

Kendler K S, Prescott C A 1997 A population-based twin study of alcohol abuse and dependence: modelling gender differences. American Journal of Medical Genetics (Neuropsychiatric Genetics) 74(6): 574

Kendler K S, Neale M C, Kessler R C, Heath A C, Eaves L J 1992 The genetic epidemiology of phobias in women: the interrelationship of agoraphobia, social phobia, situational phobia and simple phobia. Archives of General Psychiatry 49: 273–281

Kendell R E, Zealley A K 1993 Companion to psychiatric studies, 5th edn. Churchill Livingstone, Edinburgh

Kingston H M 1989 ABC of clinical genetics. British Medical Association, London

Kringlen E 1967 Heredity and social factors in schizophrenic twins: an epidemiological clinical study. In: Romano J (ed) The origins of schizophrenia. Excerpta Medical Foundation, Amsterdam

Kringlen E 1990 Genetic aspects of schizophrenia with special emphasis on twin research. In: Kringlen E (ed) Etiology of mental disorders. Department of Psychiatry, University of Oslo, p 63

Lenzinger E, Neumeister A, Praschak-Rieder N et al 1997 Association study of seasonal affective disorder and receptor genes of serotonin neurotransmission. American Journal of Medical Genetics 74(6): 590

Luxenburger H 1928 Vorlaufiger Bericht uber psychiatrische Sereinnuntersuchungen an Zwillingen. Z. Ges. Neurol. Psychiat., 116: 297–347 In: Holmes D 1991. Abnormal psychology. Harper Collins, New York

McClearn J E, Hofer S M 1997 Gender differences in heritability of alcohol use in octogenarian and nonagenarian twins. American Journal of Medical Genetics (Neuropsychiatric Genetics) 74(6): 574

McGuffin P, Katz R, Rutherford J 1991 Nature, nurture and depression: a twin study. Psychological Medicine 21(2): 329–335

Madden P A F, Heath A C, Bucholz K K et al 1997 Tolerance to alcohol and familial co-aggregation of lifetime cigarette smoking and alcohol dependence in twins. American Journal of Medical Genetics 74(6): 575

Murray R B, Huelskoetter M M W 1991 Pschiatric mental health nursing – giving emotional care, 3rd edn. Appleton & Lange, Norwalk

Murray R M, McGuffin P 1993 Genetic aspects of psychiatric disorders. In: Kendell R E, Zealley A K Companion to psychiatric studies, 5th edn. Churchill Livingstone, Edinburgh, p 227–261

Noyes R, Clancy J, Crowe R, Hoenk P R, Slymen D J 1978 The familial prevalence of anxiety neurosis. Archives of General Psychiatry 35: 1057–1059

Owen M J, McGuffin P 1992 The molecular genetics of schizophrenia (editorial). British Medical Journal 305: 664–665

Owen M J, McGuffin P 1997 Genetics and psychiatry (editorial). British Journal of Psychiatry 171: 201–202

Portin P, Alanen Y O 1997 A critical review of genetic studies of schizophrenia. I. Epidemiological and brain studies. Acta Psychiatrica Scandinavica 95: 1–5

Rose N D B (ed) 1994 Essential psychiatry, 2nd edn. Blackwell Scientific, London

Rose R J, Viken R J, Kaprio J, Koskenvuo M 1997 Use and abuse of alcohol in late adolescence: genetic dispositions interact with socioregional contexts. American Journal of Medical Genetics (Neuropsychiatric Genetics) 74(6): 577–578

Rosenthal D 1961 Sex distribution and the severity of illness among samples of schizophrenic twins. Journal of Psychiatric Research 1: 26–36

Salokangas R K R 1983 Prognostic implications of the sex of schizophrenic patients. British Journal of Psychiatry 142: 145–151

Seeman M V 1986 Current outcome in schizophrenia: women vs men. Acta Psychiatrica Scandinavica 73: 609–617

Sherrington R, Bynjolfsson J, Petursson H et al 1988 Localization of a susceptibility locus for schizophrenia on chromosome 5. Nature 336: 164–167

Simpson S G, MacKinnon D F, McInnis MG, McMahon F T, DePaulo J R 1997 Variation in suicide risk among bipolar families. American Journal of Medical Genetics (Neuropsychiatric Genetics) 74(6): 592

Szasz T 1976 Schizophrenia – the sacred symbols of psychiatry. British Journal of Psychiatry 129: 308–316

Torgensen S 1983 Genetic factors in anxiety disorders. Archives of General Psychiatry 40: 1085–1089

Tsuang M T, Gilbertson M W, Faraone S V 1991 The genetics of schizophrenia – current knowledge and future directions. Schizophrenia Research 4: 157–171

Tsuang M T, Lyons M J, Faraone S V 1990 Heterogeneity of schizophrenia: conceptual models and analytic strategies. British Journal of Psychiatry 156: 17–26

Wei J, Xu H M, Hemmings G P 1993 Studies on neurochemical heterogeneity in healthy parents of schizophrenic patients. Schizophrenia Research 10: 173–178

Xian H, True W, Eisen S A et al 1997 Evidence for a common genetic contribution to nicotine dependence and alcohol dependence. American Journal of Medical Genetics (Neuropsychiatric Genetics) 74(6): 578

Zerbin-Rudin E 1972 Genetic research and the theory of schizophrenia. International Journal of Mental Health 1: 42–62

6

Immune mechanisms and mental illness

Key Points

- Psychological stress and mental illness can compromise immune activity
- Immune activity can directly influence brain function
- In untreated depression, cellular immune activity seems to be reduced
- The therapeutic effects of antidepressants may be explained by the link between prostaglandin synthesis, reduced cellular immunity and depression
- Schizophrenia may have an autoimmune basis
- There is evidence of immune system activation with reduced activity of suppressor cells in schizophrenia
- Inconsistencies exist in the association between viral agents such as influenza and the development of schizophrenia
- Other environmental factors such as exorphins may be implicated in the pathogenesis of schizophrenia
- Although no specific viral agent has been identified there is generalised immunological dysfunction associated with chronic fatigue syndrome (CFS)
- Psychological factors and stress contribute to the development of CFS
- Individuals with AIDS may manifest a variety of mental health problems, most notably AIDS dementia complex
- AIDS dementia complex seems to develop as a result of immune activation in the brain and the production of neurotoxins
- AIDS dementia complex is not due to invasion of neurones by HIV-1
- The speed of progression and symptoms associated with AIDS dementia complex vary from individual to individual
- As survival times lengthen, the development of AIDS dementia complex may increase

In recent years, research into psychoneuroimmunology, i.e. the study of the interrelationship between the nervous system, immune system and the development of neurological and mental health problems, has grown immensely. It is over a decade since Ader (1981) provided a review of the evidence that complex interactions occurred between the brain and the immune system. Current research seems to point towards bidirectional communication between the nervous and immune systems (Altman 1997, Dunn 1995). This suggests that each modulates the other. There now appears to be general agreement that psychological stress and mental illness can compromise the immune system and, conversely, that components of the immune system can directly influence brain function. This chapter aims to consider how the immune system and the nervous system are involved in the development of mental health problems and how psychoemotional disturbance may affect the immune system. In addition, chronic fatigue syndrome (CFS) and the effect of human immunodeficiency virus (HIV) are also considered.

THE IMMUNE SYSTEM: THE ESSENTIAL COMPONENTS

The major function of the immune system is to recognise 'self' from 'nonself'. This is vitally important if a response to potentially harmful 'non-self' substances (antigenic substances) is to be mounted. In this sense immunity is said to be specific; this means that a specific response involving the production of specific cells or protein molecules to destroy a particular antigen is activated. Only a brief overview of the immune system can be provided in this chapter. For a fuller review it is suggested that Roitt (1997) is consulted.

The immune system is a highly complex system involving various white blood cells (including macrophages, T-lymphocytes and B-lymphocytes and natural killer cells) and the release of soluble chemical mediators called cytokines. The immune response essentially involves two different types of responses:

- cellular (cell-mediated) immunity
- humoral (antibody-mediated) immunity.

Humoral immunity involves the activation of B-lymphocytes in response to a foreign antigen, resulting in the growth and differentiation of B-cells into antibody (immunoglobulin)-producing plasma cells. In essence, the definition of an antigen is any molecule or microorganism that produces an antibody. Five classes of antibodies exist and are designated as IgG, IgA, IgM, IgD and IgE. Antibodies when bound to a microbe have several effects (Roitt 1997):

- activation of the classical complement pathway
- activation of phagocyctic cells
- act as opsonins and enhance phagocytosis.

Cellular immunity involves the formation of sensitised lymphocytes (T-cells). Only the particular T-cell 'programmed' to respond to a specific antigen will become sensitised and be activated. Such lymphocytes are called T-cells because unlike B-cells they differentiate within the thymus gland. The process of T-cell sensitisation involves a complex interaction with macrophages. Macrophages phagocytose the antigen and then on

Table 6.1   T-cell subtypes (selected)

T-cell subtype	Role in cellular immunity
Helper T-cells (CD4)	Induce antibody production (by the secretion of B-cell differentiation factor) Stimulate proliferation of cytotoxic (killer) T-cells and 'supressor' T-cells (by secretion of interleukin-2)
Supressor T-cells (CD8)	Inhibit cytotoxic (killer) T-cells and production of antibodies by B-cells
Cytotoxic (killer) T-cells	Destroy antigens directly (by release of lymphotoxin) and indirectly (by the secretion of other lymphokines, e.g. macrophage activating factor)
Delayed hypersensitivity T-cells	Secrete several lymphokines and are important in hypersensitivity (allergy)
Memory T-cells	Recognise original antigens
Amplifier T-cells	Stimulate exaggerated activity of helper T-cells, supressor T-cells and proliferation of plasma (differentiated B-cells) cells

the surface of the macrophage the partially digested antigen is presented to the T-cell for recognition. Sensitisation of the T-cell results in proliferation of several types of T-cells (see Table 6.1). An effective immune system requires a balance between helper and suppressor T-cells.

Cytokines are soluble factors secreted by macrophages, helper T-cells, cytotoxic killer cells and natural killer cells. Several cytokines have been isolated. Examples of these are interferons (secreted by natural killer cells and cytotoxic killer cells), interleukin-1 (secreted by macrophages) and interleukin-2 (secreted by helper T-cells). In addition to their important role in mediating cellular and humoral immune responses, circulating cytokines, by gaining access to the central nervous system, also act as neuromodulators thus influencing the neuroendocrine and behavioural responses to 'infection' and providing a 'unique integrative role between the immune system and brain function' (Leonard 1995, p 116).

IMMUNE FUNCTION AND DEPRESSION

It seems that in untreated depressed patients the lymphocyte response to allergens (as assessed by stimulation studies of peripheral blood lymphocytes) is depressed (Kronfol et al 1983), suggesting depressed cellular immune activity. Furthermore, in patients hospitalised with depression a 50% reduction in natural killer cell cytotoxicity has been observed (Irwin et al 1990). Changes in neutrophil phagocytosis have also been investigated. In depressed patients before treatment, the phagocyctosis response is significantly impaired but this returns to normal following effective treatment with antidepressants (Leonard 1995, O'Neill & Leonard 1990).

An alteration in the immune response following severe physical trauma has been well established and this has been attributed to an associated increase in serum cortisol and catecholamines and the release of prostaglandins from the damaged tissue. However, although cortisol levels are raised in depressed patients, there appears to be no evidence to suggest that it is the rise in cortisol level that leads to the impaired lymphocyte response. Lowering of the immunological competence in depressed patients was not found to be associated with the plasma cortisol concentration (Kronfol et al 1985) or to the urinary free cortisol excretion (Kronfol et al 1986).

The subnormal phagocytic response in depressed patients does not appear to be associated with changes in immunoglobulins, plasma calcium or complement, but may be due to elevated prostaglandin E_2 (Leonard

---

Case study 6.1

John is a 60-year-old business man who had run his own printing company for the past 20 years. Over this time he had slowly developed the company into an extremely large one that had large contracts with a number of publishing companies. Over the past four to five years he had become increasingly stressed and pressurised at work and at the same time his wife had suffered periods of ill health. Four years ago he developed severe rheumatoid arthritis in multiple joints, particularly affecting his wrists, hands and feet. Over the past four years John had required two separate operations on his hands and then on his feet to correct developing deformities and to reduce the pain he was experiencing. Over the same period he had received regular steroid injections to different joints to relieve his pain. Over this entire period he was in constant pain and found that he was no longer able to play golf, walk any distance or do any of the exercises that he used to do.

Over the past four months John has developed symptoms of a depressive illness with symptoms of low mood, tearfulness, feelings of hopelessness, poor sleep, poor concentration and reduced appetite. He had been referred one month previously and during the consultation spent time talking about his recent business problems, which had resulted in him taking out a further business loan. He was also having problems installing a new printing press. He felt that the business was about to collapse and that he was going to lose his house and possessions. As a result of this initial meeting, John was able, with his wife, to discuss with his partner the future of the business. He decided to take early retirement from the business and sell out to the partner.

John was started on antidepressants and admitted to hospital shortly afterwards. Over the following week his depressive illness began to lift and he expressed amazement that the joint pain had completely disappeared. The inflammatory subcutaneous skin nodules which had been a feature of his rheumatoid arthritis over the past four years also began to disappear. The levels of rheumatoid factor in his blood fell dramatically and he was able to walk long distances with no pain. The rheumatologist who had seen him over the past four years expressed considerable surprise at the complete remission of John's illness. John began to feel much happier, was sleeping better and was looking forward to his retirement.

1995). Raised concentrations of prostaglandins E_1 and E_2 have been demonstrated in depressed patients (Calabrese et al 1986) and a hypothesis has been suggested that the changes in cellular immunity may be due to the increased synthesis of prostaglandins of the E series (Calabrese et al 1986). Prostaglandins of the E series do influence the release of central nervous system (CNS) neurotransmitters and it is of interest that lithium, tricyclic antidepressants and monoamine oxidase inhibitors inhibit the synthesis of prostaglandin E. This may provide the link between the imbalance in neurotransmitter hypothesis of depression and the therapeutic effects of antidepressant drugs.

The link between alteration in the immune response and symptoms of depression is still not entirely clear (Weisse 1992). The evidence so far is derived mostly from animal models and in vitro studies, and how these relate fully to human experience is not clear. Furthermore, how far the reduced immune competence is associated with a greater risk of additional disease in depressed patients or accounts for some of the physical and emotional experiences of depressed patients still needs to be investigated more fully.

IMMUNE FUNCTION AND SCHIZOPHRENIA

Attention has been focused on the link between direct or indirect alterations of the immune system and the pathogenesis of schizophrenia. Investigations into the interaction of antibodies against brain structures, altered functions of the cellular and humoral immune systems and cytokines in blood and cerebrospinal fluid have been conducted (Muüller & Ackenheil 1995).

Studies of immunoglobulin concentrations have provided inconsistent results. Increased levels of IgA and IgM have been reported (Legros et al 1985, Pulkkinen & Soininvaara 1985). Earlier studies demonstrated an increase in IgG but this was not reproduced in later studies (Roos et al 1985). In hospitalised patients with chronic schizophrenia, decreased levels of IgA, IgM and IgG have been reported (Muüller & Ackenheil 1995).

An increase in the amount of activated B-cells in patients with schizophrenia compared to patients with depression and normal controls has been reported (Muüller & Ackenheil 1995). In addition, an increased production of peripheral autoantibodies has also been demonstrated (Spivak et al 1991).

Changes in the cellular immune system have been studied extensively, particularly T-cells and the T cell subpopulation. Elevated helper T-cells (CD4) have been demonstrated in patients receiving neuroleptic drugs (Henneberg et al 1990) and those without neuroleptic medication (Muüller et al 1991). Elevation in the helper (CD4) cell:supressor (CD8) cell ratio has also been demonstrated and this is due largely to the increase in amount of helper cells (Muüller et al 1991).

The increase in helper cells may imply persistent immune activation due to reduced suppressor cell function. Such a reduced activity of suppressor cells has been demonstrated in the sera of patients with schizophrenia (Muüller & Ackenheil 1995), supporting the hypothesis that schizophrenia may have an autoimmune basis. In addition, the function of suppressor cells seems to be genetically determined and the reduced suppressor cell activity might point to a genetically determined alteration in the immune system as the basis for the development of schizophrenia (Muüller & Ackenheil 1995). This is further supported by the demonstration of reduced serum levels of interleukin-2 (IL-2) and increased interleukin-2 receptors in patients with schizophrenia (Muüller & Ackenheil 1995). Interleukin-2 is vital for activation of suppressor cells. Cytokines (e.g. IL-2), which are actively transported into the CNS, play a key role in the immune activation and have a strong influence on dopaminergic, noradrenergic and serotonergic neurotransmission (Muüller & Ackenheil 1998).

It seems that there is activation of the immune system in a high proportion of patients with schizophrenia. This activation is consistent with both the autoimmune and viral hypotheses of the pathogenesis of schizophrenia.

The development of the viral hypothesis is based on the known excess of births of schizophrenic individuals during the winter and spring months (Franzek & Beckmann 1996) and the possible association between influenza epidemics and the birthdates of schizophrenic patients. The link is that maternal viral infection occurring at a vulnerable period in fetal brain development may result in brain abnormalities leading to schizophrenia in later life. Several epidemiological studies have suggested that maternal exposure to influenza, particularly the A2 influenza virus during the second trimester, is a risk factor for schizophrenia (Adams et al 1993, Takei et al 1994, 1996a). Indeed it has been suggested that exposure to the influenza virus may lead to the development of morphological abnormalities of the brain of the kind frequently reported in schizophrenic patients (Takei et al 1996b).

However, inconsistencies exist in the results. So far the association between prenatal influence and an increased risk of schizophrenia in adulthood has been found only in population-based data (Cannon et al 1996). When comparing a group of women who were known to have been exposed to influenza with a group not exposed, no association was demonstrated (Cannon et al 1996). Similar findings have been reported from Western Australia (Morgan et al 1997) and among Surinamese and Dutch Antillean immigrants to the Netherlands (Selten et al 1998).

It has been reported that Borna disease virus (BDV) may be associated with schizophrenia and depression (Rott et al 1985). A significantly higher proportion of anti-BDV antibody has been found in Japanese (Iwahashi et al 1997) and Chinese schizophrenic patients from Taiwan and their carers and health care workers (Chen et al 1999). The route of transmission of BDV is unclear and the role of BDV in the pathogenesis of schizophrenia requires further study.

It may be the case that in time other environmental factors may become implicated in the immunological basis of schizophrenia. Exorphins (proteins derived from the process of digestion that act as biological modulators) may be one such factor. De Santis et al (1997) reported that introducing a gluten-free diet to a 33-year-old patient with pre-existing schizophrenia who had coeliac disease resulted in a disappearance of psychiatric symptoms and a return to normal perfusion of the frontal cortex.

IMMUNE SYSTEM AND CHRONIC FATIGUE SYNDROME (CFS)

CFS has been described as 'a genuine but poorly understood illness' (Krupp & Pollina 1996). 'Fatigue' as an established symptom is well recognised, although there appears to be a spectrum from 'normal fatigue' on the one hand to the fatigue associated with CFS on the other (Wessely et al 1998). Community surveys in Europe and North America using slightly different definitions of 'fatigue' indicate that this symptom is very common, occurring in up to 33% of men and 42% of women (Lewis & Wessely 1992).

The understanding of CFS has been troubled by inconsistencies in the diagnostic criteria applied. Attempts have been made to standardise the criteria. Fukuda et al (1994) have suggested that 'fatigue' in the context of CFS must be of new onset, not be due to ongoing exertion, not be alleviated by rest and result in substantial reduction of previous occupational, educational, social or personal activities. The Oxford Criteria (Sharpe et al 1991, Wessely et al 1998) identify specific criteria for the diagnosis of

---

Box 6.1   The Oxford Criteria used for the diagnosis of CFS (Sharpe et al 1991, by permission of Royal Society of Medicine Press; Wessely et al 1998, by permission of Oxford University Press)

Maximum duration 6 months
Functional impairment: disabling
Cognitive or neuropsychiatric symptoms: mental fatigue required
Other symptoms: not specific
New onset required
Medical exclusions: known physical causes of fatigue
Psychiatric exclusions: psychosis, bipolar, eating disorders, organic brain disease

CFS (Box 6.1). With regard to individual experiences, in addition to fatigue, mild memory impairment and increased reaction times may be experienced, along with sleep disturbance, muscle aches and perceived muscle weakness.

The aetiology of the syndrome was first considered to be a viral infection. No specific virus has been identified and elevated antibody titres to a range of viral agents have been demonstrated, including antibodies to herpes, measles virus and cytomegalovirus. While a direct link between a specific virus and CFS has not been established there is nevertheless generalised immunological dysfunction associated with CFS. Wessely et al (1998) state that 'CFS is a reality after certain infections' (p 182), with Epstein-Barr, Q-fever, toxoplasmosis and cytomegalovirus being the most likely causative agents.

Most studies suggest a mild disturbance in humoral activity, featuring elevation in B-cells and B-cell subsets (Tirelli et al 1994). A more consistent finding in CFS is disturbance of the cellular immune system. Defects in and reduced numbers of natural killer cells have been observed (Krupp & Pollina 1996). T-cell abnormalities include increased activation of suppressor (CD8) cells and depressed response to mitogenic stimulation (Straus et al 1993).

Immune abnormalities are often very subtle and again are identified in some cases only in vitro. Whether or not the immune abnormalities demonstrated in CFS are a primary or secondary phenomenon remains to be established. Moreover, how specific these immune abnormalities are to CFS is not clear. As identified earlier in the chapter, many of the immune changes are also found in affective disorders, and disorders of affect are a feature of CFS. Indeed, while there is evidence of some abnormalities of the immune system the findings are inconsistent and there does not seem to be a strong correlation between immunological dysfunction and clinical condition (Wessely et al 1998).

Estimates of the frequency of mental illness associated with CFS are as high as 52–86% for lifetime psychiatric illness (Krupp & Pollina 1996). In a series of studies using the Depression Inventory Scale, the majority of subjects whose main complaint was chronic fatigue were found to be depressed (Manu et al 1988). However, while a large number of individuals who experience CFS also satisfy criteria for the diagnosis of a psychiatric condition, CFS is not associated with any single psychiatric disorder (Wessely et al 1998). Indeed, Wessely et al (1998) suggest that there may be a stronger link between anxiety disorders and CFS than with depression.

Essentially the underlying aetiology of CFS remains unclear. It has been suggested that hormonal dysfunction centred around the hypothalamic-pituitary-adrenal axis might be responsible for the physical and psychological problems associated with CFS (Demitrack 1994).

Dysfunction of the hypothalamus could explain the symptoms of fatigue, fever and appetite changes, and decreases in cortisol levels have been reported in CFS, but the picture is not clear and further research in this area is required before any firm conclusions can be reached. Discussion of stress, chronic fatigue and the immune system is developed further in Chapter 10.

Psychological factors and stress contribute to the development of CFS, suggesting that psychological vulnerability and coping style are important in CFS. As a unifying approach, Krupp & Pollina (1996) suggest that 'an individual with elevated stress and poor coping skills has associated immune pertubations, which in conjunction with an external insult such as a viral infection, lead to prolonged illness' (p 159).

AIDS DEMENTIA AND OTHER AIDS-RELATED NEUROPSYCHIATRIC DISORDERS

It has been reported that HIV-related neuropsychiatric syndromes occur in approximately 30% of adults and 50% of children with AIDS (Lipton & Gendelman 1996). Four broad categories of neuropsychiatric problems have been identified (Keltner et al 1998):

- psychological distress related to fatal illness
- neuropsychiatric complications of the primary HIV brain infection
- neuropsychiatric complications of secondary opportunistic brain infections or secondary brain tumours
- nervous system complications from medical therapies.

AIDS results from infection by HIV. HIV-1 virus and the related HIV-2 virus have been isolated from various body fluids of individuals with AIDS. HIV-1 and HIV-2 are members of the lentivirus subfamily of the human retrovirus. AIDS is distinguished from HIV infection by the occurrence of opportunistic infection such as atypical pneumonia due to the microorganism *Pneumocyctis carinii* or AIDS-related malignancies, for example Kaposi's sarcoma or a significant decrease in the helper (CD4) cell:suppressor (CD8) cell ratio. Individuals typically develop a range of physical symptoms including fatigue, weight loss, anorexia and malaise. However, due to the depressed immune activity atypical viral, fungal and bacterial infections can occur in the brain leading to overt neuropsychiatric problems.

HIV-1 enters the brain by crossing the blood–brain barrier. Significant brain infection may be delayed until the development of AIDS (Portegies 1994). Keltner et al (1998) describe three general stages:

- entry into CNS macrophages
- invasion and replication within brain macrophages

- production of neurotoxic substances by CNS macrophages and astrocytes, leading to neuronal damage or death.

At present the timing of and mechanism for HIV-1 infection of the CNS still needs to be determined fully. There is no direct evidence that HIV-1 invades the neurone (Lipton & Gendelman 1996). The neuropathogenesis of CNS viral infection centres around the infection of CNS macrophages and microglial cells, leading to immune activation in the brain (Lipton 1997, Zheng & Gendelman 1997). HIV binds to membrane-bound receptors on the macrophage, and the complex then enters the macrophage. Low levels of neurotoxins are then produced by the macrophage and released into the local extracellular environment. HIV is inserted into the macrophage genome and replication occurs.

This process results in the production of large amounts of various neurotoxins that stimulate adjacent astrocytes to produce additional substances, including cytokines and interleukins (Lipton 1997, Zheng & Gendelman 1997). Each chemical changes the microenvironment of the brain profoundly. Neuronal death or diminished neuronal function as a result of decreased numbers of dendrites is the end result, with proliferation of macrophages and activation of astrocytes.

Individuals with and without dementia have HIV in their brain tissue and seemingly the viral load does not predict the risk of developing dementia (Johnson et al 1996). HIV infection also damages white matter within the CNS, although the mechanism for this is not yet established. It has been proposed that HIV triggers an autoimmune phenomenon similar to multiple sclerosis or that cytotoxic substances produced as a result of HIV infection may damage oligodendrocytes (Keltner et al 1998).

As a result of the primary infection of the brain with HIV, secondary infection with opportunistic pathogens and secondary brain tumours, individuals with AIDS may manifest a variety of mental health problems (see Box 6.2), most notably *AIDS dementia complex*.

AIDS dementia complex is a term that describes a variable collection of cognitive, motor and behavioural abnormalities in patients with AIDS (Keltner et al 1996). Of those infected with HIV who develop AIDS, 60% may also develop AIDS dementia (Portegies 1994), with dementia being the presenting problem in some cases (Rabins 1996). Of those who die from AIDS, 90% demonstrate neuropathological alterations in the brain,

---

Box 6.2   Mental health problems associated with HIV infection and AIDS

Adjustment disorders: for example anxiety, panic attacks or depressed mood
Disorders of mood: unipolar or bipolar affective disorders
Organic mental disorders: AIDS dementia complex, tumour-associated diseases
Delirium

suggesting that as survival times lengthen with improved drug cocktails, the prevalence of AIDS dementia may increase (Keltner et al 1998).

The clinical progression of AIDS dementia has been divided into early, middle and late stages, with the speed of progression and the symptoms varying from individual to individual. Early symptoms include difficulties with memory, concentration and conceptualisation. With progressing dementia, individuals may develop apraxia, dysarthria and frontal lobe dysfunction (Keltner et al 1998). No AIDS dementia-specific abnormalities have been identified using brain imaging techniques or at postmortem. Indeed the variable pathological findings do not correlate with the severity of the disease.

No specific region of the brain is most affected. Variable degrees of cortical atrophy and ventriculomegaly are present. Microscopically, some cases have no abnormal manifestations while in other patients microglial nodules and proliferation of individual neuroglial cells is evident.

CONCLUSION

The introduction to this chapter identified that the interaction between the CNS and the immune system is both highly complex and bidirectional. With the advance of improved immunological techniques and the isolation of more specific immunological markers, the interplay between immune system activity and the development and progression of mental health problems will in time be understood more fully. For the moment specific mental health conditions associated with changes in immunological activity have been discussed in this chapter. In Chapter 10 the link between stress and the immune system is developed further.

REFERENCES

Adams W, Kendell R E, Hare E H, Munk-Jorgensen P 1993 Epidemiological evidence that maternal influenza contributes to the aetiology of schizophrenia. British Journal of Psychiatry 163: 522–534
Ader R (ed) 1981 Psychoneuroimmunology. Academic Press, New York
Altman F 1997 Where is the 'neuro' in psychoneuroimmunology? Brain Behaviour and Immunity 11: 1–8
Calabrese J, Skwereer R G, Barna B et al 1986 Depression, immunocompetence and prostaglandins of the E series. Psychiatry Research 17: 44–47
Cannon M, Cotter D, Coffey V P et al 1996 Prenatal exposure to the 1957 influenza epidemic and adult schizophrenia: a follow-up study. British Journal of Psychiatry 168: 368–371
Chen C H, Chiu Y L, Wei F C et al 1999 High seroprevalence of Borna virus infection in schizophrenic patients, family members and mental health workers in Taiwan. Molecular Psychiatry 4: 33–38
De Santis A, Addolorato G, Romito A et al 1997 Schizophrenia symptoms and SPECT abnormalities in a coeliac patient: regression after a gluten-free diet. Journal of Internal Medicine 242: 421–423

Demitrack M A 1994 Chronic fatigue syndrome: a disease of the hypothalamic-pituitary-adrenal axis? Annals of Medicine 26: 1–5

Dunn A J 1995 Psychoneuroimmunology: introduction and general perspectives. In: Leonard B E, Miller K (eds) Stress, the immune system and psychiatry. Wiley, Chichester, p 1

Franzek E, Beckmann H 1996 Gene–environment interaction in schizophrenia: season-of-birth effect reveals etiologically different subgroups. Psychopathology 29: 14–26

Fukuda K, Straus S E, Hickie I, Sharpe M C, Dobbins J G, Komaroff A 1994 The chronic fatigue syndrome: a comprehensive approach to its definition and study. Annals of Internal Medicine 121: 953–959

Henneberg A, Riedl B, Dumke H O, Kornhuber H H 1990 T-lymphocyte subpopulations in schizophrenic patients. European Archives of Psychology & Neurological Sciences 239: 283–284

Irwin M, Patterson T, Smith T L et al 1990 Reduction in immune function in life stress and depression. Biological Psychiatry 27: 22–30

Iwahashi K, Watanabe M, Nakamura K et al 1997 Clinical investigation of the relationship between Borna disease virus (BDV) infection and schizophrenia in 67 patients in Japan. Acta Psychiatrica Scandinavica 96: 412–415

Johnson R T, Glass J D, McArthur J C, Chesebro B W 1996 Quantitation of human immunodeficiency virus in brains of demented and non-demented patients with acquired immunodeficiency syndrome. Annals of Neurology 39: 392–395

Keltner N L, Folks D G, Palmer C A, Powers R E 1998 Psychobiological foundations of psychiatric care. Mosby, St Louis

Kronfol Z, Silva J, Greden J, Gardner R, Carroll B J 1983 Impaired lymphocyte function in depressive illness. Life Sciences 33: 241–242

Kronfol Z, Nasrallah H A, Chapman S, House J D 1985 Depression, cortisol metabolism and lymphocytopenia. Journal of Affective Disorders 9: 169–173

Kronfol Z, House J D, Siolva J, Greden J, Carroll B J 1986 Depression, urinary free cortisol excretion and lymphocyte function. British Journal of Psychiatry 148: 70–73

Krupp L B, Pollina D 1996 Neuroimmune and neuropsychiatric aspects of chronic fatigue syndrome. Advances in Neuroimmunology 6: 155–167

Legros S, Mendlewicz J, Wybran J 1985 Immunoglobulins, autoantibodies and other serum protein fractions in psychiatric disorders. European Archives of Psychiatry and Neurological Sciences 235: 9–11

Leonard B E 1995 Stress and the immune system: immunological aspects of depressive illness. In: Leonard B E, Miller K (eds) Stress, the immune system and psychiatry. Wiley, Chichester, p 113–136

Lewis G, Wessely S 1992 The epidemiology of fatigue: more questions than answers. Journal of Epidemiology and Community Health 46: 92–97

Lipton S A 1997 Neuropathogenesis of acquired immunodeficiency syndrome dementia. Current Opinion in Neurology 10: 247–253

Lipton S A, Gendelman E 1996 Dementia associated with acquired immunodeficiency syndrome. In: Flier J S, Underhill L H. Seminars of the Beth Israel Hospital. New England Journal of Medicine 332: 934–940

Manu P, Matthews D A, Lane T J 1988 The mental health of patients with a chief complaint of chronic fatigue. Archives of Internal Medicine 148: 2213–2217

Morgan V, Castle D, Page A et al 1997 Influenza epidemics and incidence of schizophrenia, affective disorders and mental retardation in Western Australia: no evidence of major effect. Schizophrenia Research 26: 25–39

Muüller N, Ackenheil M 1995 The immune system and schizophrenia. In: Leonard B E Miller K 1995 (eds) Stress, the immune system and psychiatry. Wiley, Chichester, p 137

Muüller N, Ackenheil M 1998 Psychoneuroimmunology and the cytokine action in the CNS: implications for psychiatric disorders. Progress in Neuro-Psychopharmacology and Biological Psychiatry 22: 1–33

Muüller N, Ackenheil M, Hof schuster E, Mempel W, Eckstein R 1991 Cellular immunity in schizophrenic patients before and during neuroleptic therapy. Psychiatry Research 37: 147–160

O'Neill B, Leonard B E 1990 Abnormal zymosin-induced neutrophil chemiluminescence as a marker of depression. Journal of Affective Disorders 19: 269–272

Portegies P 1994 AIDS dementia complex: a review. Journal of Acquired Immune Deficiency Syndrome 7 (suppl 2): S38–S49

Pulkkinen E, Soininvaara O 1985 Immunoglobulins in schizophrenics and prediction of need for hospital care. Acta Psychiatrica Scandinavica 72: 133–138

Rabins P V 1996 Dementia as a symptom of HIV disease. Lancet 347: 769–770

Roitt I M 1997 Roitt's essential immunology, 9th edn. Blackwell Science, Oxford

Roos R P, Davis K, Meltzer H Y 1985 Immunoglobulin studies in patients with psychiatric diseases. Archives of General Psychiatry 42: 124–128

Rott R, Herzog S, Fleischer B et al 1985 Detection of serum antibodies to Borna disease virus in patients with psychiatric disorders. Science 228: 755–756

Selten J P, Slaets J, Kahn R 1998 Prenatal exposure to influenza and schizophrenia in Surinamese and Dutch Antillean immigrants to the Netherlands. Schizophrenia Research 30: 101–103

Sharpe M C, Archard L C, Banatvala J E et al 1991 A report: chronic fatigue syndrome: guidelines for research. Journal of the Royal Society of Medicine 84: 118–121

Spivak B, Marguerite R, Brandon J et al 1991 Cold agglutinin autoantibodies in psychiatric patients: their relationship to diagnosis and pharmacological treatment. American Journal of Psychiatry 148: 244–247

Straus S E, Fritz S, Dale J K, Gould B, Strober W 1993 Lymphocyte phenotype and function in chronic fatigue syndrome. Journal of Clinical Immunology 13: 30–40

Takei N, Sham P, O'Callaghan E, Murray G K, Glover G, Murray R M 1994 Prenatal exposure to influenza and the development of schizophrenia: is the effect confined to females? American Journal of Psychiatry 151: 117–119

Takei N, Mortensen P B, Klaening U et al 1996a Relationship between in utero exposure to influenza epidemics and risk of schizophrenia in Denmark. Biological Psychiatry 40: 817–824

Takei N, Lewis S, Jones P, Harvey I, Murray R M 1996b Prenatal exposure to influenza and increased cerebrospinal fluid spaces in schizophrenia. Schizophrenia Bulletin 22: 521–534

Tirelli U, Marotta G, Improta S, Pinto A 1994 Immunological abnormalities in patients with chronic fatigue syndrome. Scandinavian Journal of Immunology 40: 601–608

Weisse C S 1992 Depression and immunocompetence: a review of the literature. Psychological Bulletin 111: 475–489

Wessely S, Hotopf M, Sharp M 1998 Chronic fatigue and its syndromes. Oxford University Press, Oxford

Zheng J, Gendelman H E 1997 The HIV-1 associated dementia complex; a metabolic encephalopathy fueled by viral replication in mononuclear phagocytes. Current Opinion in Neurology 10: 19–25

7

Nutrition and mental health

Key Points

- Mental illness can lead to malnutrition, and nutritional factors may lead to mental health problems
- Carbohydrate consumption has an effect on mood
- It is possible for either weight loss or weight gain to occur during episodes of depression
- There is a relationship between folate deficiency and depression
- Essential fatty acids appear to have a role in neurotransmission and in the biology of schizophrenia
- Low 5HT increases appetite and high 5HT decreases appetite
- Cholecystokinin inhibits both feeding and gastric emptying and may be an inhibitory factor in anorexia nervosa
- Micronutrient deficiencies can produce features associated with mental health problems
- Vitamin B1 deficiency can lead to emotional fatigue and physical weakness
- Vitamin B6 deficiency can lead to fatigue, nervousness, irritability, depression, insomnia and walking difficulties
- Alcohol abuse can lead to both mineral and vitamin deficiencies
- Hypersensitivity reactions to ingested food substances produce symptoms of mental illness

The relationship between mental health and nutrition can be dealt with from two perspectives. One perspective examines mental illness as a cause of malnutrition, and the other deals with how nutritional factors may lead to mental health problems. An array of psychosocial and environmental factors can lead an individual to adopt a diet that is nutritionally inadequate since eating and feeding behaviours are often bound up with family dynamics and may be a barometer of a family's emotional climate and parent–child interactions.

This chapter describes briefly the theories of food intake and the physiological basis of hunger and satiety. Aspects of healthy eating and the need to establish regular healthy eating habits so as to minimise the development of a maladaptive eating pattern and malnutrition are addressed and emphasis is stressed on eating as a communal event (i.e. the therapeutic value of eating). The role of some specific nutrients is discussed in relation to how behaviour and cognitive function may be affected as a consequence of nutritional deficiency and toxicity.

THEORIES ASSOCIATED WITH FOOD INTAKE AND APPETITE CONTROL

Appetite can be described as the individual's preference for food which is culturally determined and may or may not be associated with hunger. There is no doubt that the desire to eat certain foods or dishes very much depends on habits of eating, cultural indoctrination and on pleasant or unpleasant experiences associated with those particular foods. Thus the selection of a food and the desire to eat may depend very much on the smell, flavour, appearance and appeal of the food. Indeed some cultures have savoury foods designed to stimulate appetite, as epitomised by the *mazza* in Egypt, the *meze* in Greece, the *zakuska* in Russia, the *smorgasbork* in Scandinavia and the *tapas* in Spain.

The consumption of food to satisfy nutritional needs and deficiencies in the body can be described as hunger. Such hunger may be very specific to satisfy energy deficiencies, calcium or sodium deficiencies, thus influencing choice of foods to be eaten. From a physiological and biochemical perspective, several theories associated with appetite and food intake have been put forward. Some of these have been reviewed by Holmes (1986); in this review, Holmes states that at the end of the day, the individual is the ultimate arbiter of his or her own personal health behaviour and will choose what to eat and what not to eat. As early as 1898, Cannon proposed the stomach distension theory in which he stated that an empty stomach contracts causing 'hunger pangs' and distension of the stomach stops an animal or individual from feeding.

The glucostatic theory (Meyer & Bates 1951, Mayer et al 1952, Mayer 1953) refers to glucoreceptors in the hypothalamus and liver being sensitive to the rate of blood glucose utilisation with the result that feeding is stimulated or inhibited when blood glucose is low or high respectively. Kennedy (1953) proposed the lipostatic theory which deals with the control of long-term eating behaviour and suggests that some factor in blood is in dynamic equilibrium with total adipose tissue. Total adipose tissue influences hypothalamic centres and food intake. The degree of feeding varies inversely in relation to the total amount of adipose tissue.

The thermostatic theory (Brobeck 1948) suggested that some interaction exists within the hypothalamus between the system regulating body temperature and that regulating food intake. It is now well established that the act of eating and digesting food, known as the *specific dynamic action of food*, increases an individual's metabolic rate by 10–20%. Specific dynamic action of food is greatest with proteins and less when carbohydrate and fats are eaten. Harper et al (1970) proposed the aminostatic theory which deals with concentration of amino acids in blood: a high concentration of amino acids stimulates feeding.

While each of these theories is very plausible, the factors that regulate appetite and feeding behaviour are complex and encompass physiological, biochemical, sociocultural and psychological factors. The importance of understanding nutritional issues in mental health in terms of both assessment and diagnosis in clinical practice as well as from health promotion and intervention perspectives cannot be overemphasised.

EFFECTS OF NUTRITIONAL FACTORS ON MOOD AND PSYCHOSOCIAL FUNCTIONING

Studies by Benton et al (1982) in which a glucose tolerance test was given to males with no history of violence showed a relationship between mild hypoglycaemia and questionnaire measures of an aggressive tendency. Further studies by Benton et al (1987) found that there was sustained attention and better reaction to frustration in 6-year-old children who had received a glucose drink than in those children who had consumed a placebo. However, other studies by Thayer (1987) found increased tension one hour after a sugar snack. These later findings may be related to the time scale between the initial increase in blood glucose and the release of insulin. Later studies by Benton & Owen (1993) found that higher blood glucose levels were associated with lower feelings of tension.

The consumption of a sugary drink in the absence of protein and fat must be put into its true context since in practice individuals have a tendency to eat food in which all three macronutrients – carbohydrates, protein and fat – are found. This contextual basis does not change the fact that carbohydrate meals that contain little protein increase the uptake of tryptophan into the brain, resulting in increased synthesis and release of serotonin (Spring & Chiodo 1987). Since serotonergic neurones have some influence on pain, sleep and mood regulation, they may be responsible for the calming of mood following the sugary drink (Benton & Owen 1993, Spring & Chiodo 1987).

Other studies by Sullivan et al (1993) on the impact of obesity and related morbidity on perceived health and psychosocial functioning have shown that severely obese individuals reported poorer current health status, a less positive mood state and more social dysfunction than general population samples. These findings were valid for both men and women, with anxiety and depression scores being higher in severely obese women than in men. The same authors report that less social interaction was seen in the severely obese than in those with other clinical conditions where individuals had adapted to their diagnosis or handicap, such as cancer survivors (two to three years after diagnosis with no recurrence). Sullivan et al (1993) recommend the re-evaluation of impaired quality of life in severe obesity beyond the impact of medical complications.

Associated with the issue of obesity is the direction of weight change that occurs in recurrent depression as discussed by Stunkard et al (1990) who showed that there was a very high concordance between two episodes of depression and the direction and extent of weight loss. Stunkard et al (1990) demonstrated that most people who lost weight during one episode of depression also lost it during another, while most of those who gained weight during one episode of depression also gained it during another. This is supported by studies by Di Pietro et al (1992) who showed that younger men (under 55 years of age) who were depressed at baseline gained nearly 3 kg more over a follow-up period than those who were not depressed. It was noticed, however, that education modified the effect of depression on weight change, with those having fewer than 12 years of education gaining more weight with depression than those with more education. Among younger women, the authors found that depressed younger women gained slightly less weight than those who were not depressed, with those having fewer than 12 years of education gaining less weight with depression than those with more education. Among older people (over 55 years of age), both men and women who were depressed lost more weight than those who were not depressed. Thus weight gain does occur in depression and the current use of weight loss only in depression inventories (Beck et al 1961, Hamilton 1960, Zung et al 1974) is less sensitive.

THE ROLE OF FOLATE (FOLIC ACID) IN DEPRESSION

Depressive symptoms are the most common neuropsychiatric manifestation of folate deficiency (Alpert & Fava 1997). After four months on a folate deficiency diet, Herbert (1961) reported some evidence supporting the relationship between folate deficiency and depression. Further studies (Ghadirian et al 1980, Reynolds 1967) provided more evidence on the link between folic acid deficiency and depression. Reynolds (1967) found an improvement of mental state with folic acid treatment in 22 out of 26 folate-deficient epileptic patients and reported that the most notable changes seen in the patients in this study were in drive, initiative and elevation of mood. Studies by Ghadirian et al (1980) found that serum folic acid levels were significantly lower in depressed patients than in medical and other psychiatric patients and also noted that those patients with the lowest folic acid levels also obtained higher ratings on depressed mood and decreased work productivity. More recently, in their study of patients with severe folate deficiency that results in megaloblastic anaemia, Alpert & Fava (1997) report depressive symptoms as the most common. This association between folate deficiency and depression is stronger with endogenous depression (psychotic depression) than with neurotic depression (Carney et al 1990).

An important area that has been studied by several workers is the relationship of folate levels with response to antidepressant treatment. Previous studies by Carney & Sheffield (1970) showed that psychiatric patients given folic acid had reduced inpatient time, improved mood and showed better social functioning skills than those who were not given folic acid. Later studies by Coppen et al (1986) in individuals with unipolar and bipolar mood disorders indicated that administration of folic acid to patients receiving lithium prophylactically reduced the reoccurrence and duration of mood disorder symptoms.

In other investigations (Reynolds et al 1970), it was found that not only were depressed inpatients with low folate levels at admission more severely depressed than those with normal folate levels, but they also showed higher ratings of depression and neuroticism at discharge after treatment with antidepressants or tryptophan or electroconvulsive therapy (ECT) than those with normal folate levels. This is supported by more recent workers (Fava et al 1997) who found that individuals suffering from major bipolar disorder (manic depressive disorder) with low serum folate levels before the start of antidepressant therapy responded more poorly to eight weeks of therapy with the selective serotonin reuptake inhibitor (SSRI) fluoxetine at a dosage of 20 mg per day than those patients with normal folate levels. Further evidence is given by Alpert et al (1996) who demonstrated the association between red blood cell folate and response to sertraline and nortriptyline.

Other observations (Botez et al 1979, Hunter et al 1967) suggest a curvilinear relationship between folate levels and response to antidepressant therapy and that there is a therapeutic window whereby too little or too much folate supplementation does not help depressed patients, as indicated by studies showing irritability, hyperactivity, malaise and altered sleep patterns in healthy volunteers given 15 mg of folate daily.

However, there is no doubt that folate and methylfolate play an important role in depression and its treatment. Methylfolate is actively transported into the central nervous system (CNS) across the blood–brain barrier and is concentrated in synaptic regions where it participates in essential metabolic pathways (Godfrey et al 1990). Methylfolate is also detectable in cerebrospinal fluid (CSF) in concentrations three times greater than in serum (Reynolds 1979, Spector 1979).

NUTRITION AND SCHIZOPHRENIA

In their study, Ramchand et al (1992) suggest that folate deficiency does not cause schizophrenia but that deficiency in folate may be the result of both the severity and chronicity of the illness as well as the medication given to treat sufferers. Their conclusion raises the question as to whether it may be prudent to initiate folate supplementation at the time when neuroleptic management of the patient is started.

In other studies, Godfrey et al (1990) showed that a subgroup of patients with schizophrenia treated with methlyfolate showed better clinical and social recovery than a group given a placebo. The benefits of methylfolate over placebo became more significant with time, thus supporting the view that the response of the nervous system to folate may occur slowly (Reynolds 1967). It appears that the effect of folic acid on mental function, especially mood, is reinforced by the effect of S-adenosylmethionine which donates methyl groups in many of the methylation reactions in the nervous system where neurotransmitters, membrane phospholipids, proteins and nucleoproteins are involved (Godfrey et al 1990).

The role of essential fatty acids has been linked with both neural deficits and mental functioning. In their studies, Peet et al (1994) suggest that arachidonic acid is the common link in the biology of schizophrenia. Arachidonic acid is the main precursor in the synthesis of prostaglandins and, according to Barbour et al (1989), arachidonic acid acts as a second messenger in glutamatergic neurotransmission. This means that when the availability of arachidonic acid is reduced, glutamatergic neurotransmission is impaired and some evidence (Carlsson & Carlsson 1990) from postmortem studies supports the view that glutamate neurotransmitter systems are impaired in schizophrenia. These same authors have proposed that schizophrenia is a result of dopamine–glutamate imbalance and that prostaglandins are also involved in dopaminergic neurotransmission. Prostaglandins are unsaturated fatty acids with 20 carbon atoms. According to Hardy (1984), prostaglandins were a chance discovery and were first demonstrated in the 1930s when semen was found to contain a stimulant for smooth muscle. Hitherto, over 16 prostaglandins have been characterised.

Royston & Lewis (1993) have put forward a hypothesis (Fig. 7.1) that during increased arachidonic acid metabolism, free radicals are generated which cause neural deficits and other morphological abnormalities that have been identified in the brains of schizophrenic patients. A general increase in metabolism can lead to an increase in free radicals. In addition, an increase in catecholamine turnover increases free radical production. This increased free radical production or a deficiency of antioxidant enzymes (genetic or due to cofactor abnormality) can produce increased oxidative stress. The end result is neuronal dysfunction due to lipid peroxidation. Norwegian studies by Odegard (1956) and Sundby & Nyhus (1963) on the incidence of schizophrenia in ordinary seamen showed that there was a higher incidence of schizophrenia in seamen when compared

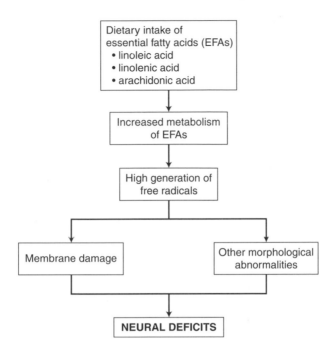

Figure 7.1 A hypothetical model that links nutrition with neural deficits and mental functioning.

with all other occupational groups. Dietary analyses revealed that the diet of seamen was high in total fat (predominantly saturated fats), accounting for 46% of ingested calories (Eggen et al 1964 cited in Christensen & Christensen 1988).

While the incidence of schizophrenia appears similar in different parts of the world, the outcome of treatment intervention is more favourable in developing countries than in industrialised countries (Sartorius et al 1978, World Health Organization 1979). This difference in response is attributed to dietary factors. Individuals in developing countries by and large consume a diet high in unsaturated fat. A high intake of unsaturated fat may benefit schizophrenic patients, possibly because essential fatty acids may be deficient in such patients (Christensen & Christensen 1988). These same authors concluded from their own studies, and the statistical association of other studies, that a high percentage of fat from vegetables, fish and seafood tended to be associated with a favourable outcome. More recently, studies by Mellor et al (1996) have supported the view that a high intake of some essential fatty acids such as eicosapentanoic acid (EPA) in normal diet is associated with less severe schizophrenic symptoms, especially positive symptoms, and may lessen the severity of tardive dyskinesia.

EATING DISORDERS

The two main eating disorders that are discussed in this chapter are anorexia nervosa and bulimia nervosa. The powerful force at work in both these disorders is the underlying distressing fear of fatness (Crisp et al 1996) which can be described as a dyslipophobia. Puri et al (1996) have given a comprehensive multifactorial aetiology of eating disorders that covers the predisposing, perpetuating and precipitating factors.

Bulimia nervosa

Bulimia nervosa refers to binge eating, which is the rapid consumption of a large amount of food in a discrete period of time (Weltzin et al 1994). There is now a growing body of evidence to support the relationship between decreased activity of serotonin 5HT in the CNS and bulimia nervosa (Weltzin et al 1994). Since 5HT is one of the neurotransmitters that modulate appetite, it has been shown experimentally in animals (Fig. 7.2) that reducing 5HT activity increases food intake while increasing 5HT activity does the reverse (Weltzin et al 1994).

L-tryptophan is the essential amino acid from which 5HT is synthesised and this amino acid is obtained naturally from the diet. The amount of 5HT synthesised in the CNS depends on the amount of tryptophan that crosses from the blood into the CNS. Competition from other amino acids for transport routes may lead to a low level of tryptophan in the CNS, resulting in reduced synthesis of 5HT (Fernstrom & Wurtman 1971, 1972).

Since 5-hydroxyindoleacetic acid (5HIAA) is a metabolite of 5HT, studies in bulimic anorexic patients have shown lower levels of 5HIAA in the

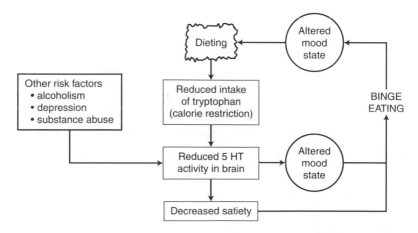

Figure 7.2 5HT activity and bulimia. Adapted from Welzin et al (1994).

CSF when compared to non-bulimic anorexic patients (Kaye et al 1984). This is supported by other investigations (Kaye at al 1990) which showed that bulimic women of normal weight without anorexia nervosa but with severe bulimic symptoms also have reduced levels of CSF 5HIAA. Jimerson et al (1992) also presented supporting evidence that showed that a subgroup of patients with severe symptoms of bulimia nervosa had decreased CSF concentrations of 5HIAA and homovallinic acid, the two being metabolites of serotonin and dopamine respectively. Acute tryptophan depletion in male non-human primates (vervet monkeys) has been found to increase aggression during competition for food

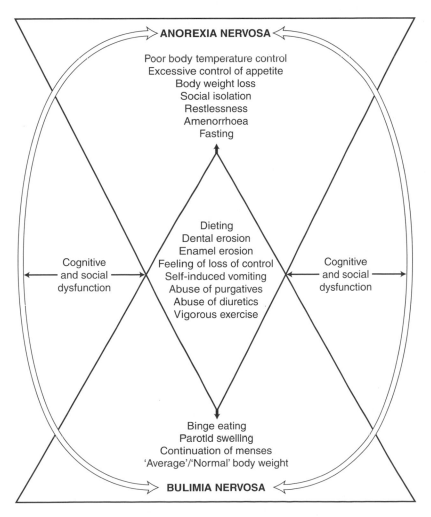

Figure 7.3 A physiological–behavioural model for anorexia and bulimia nervosa. Adapted from Meades (1993), by permission of Blackwell Science Ltd.

(Chamberlain et al 1987) while such depletion in humans has led to increased dysphoria and reduced protein intake (Young et al 1985).

The physiological manifestations of bulimia have been covered in detail by other authors (Dippel & Becknal 1987, Fairburn 1993, Hofland & Dardis 1992, Levin et al 1980, Meades 1993). What is important for health care workers is to realise the significance of the manifestations that result from self-induced vomiting, laxative abuse or diuretic abuse as discussed by the cited authors (see Fig. 7.3). Since bulimia is characterised by denial and secretiveness and the physical and metabolic problems such as weakness, fatigue and sore throat are often non-specific, it is easy to misinterpret patient problems as psychogenic unless nurses and other health care workers possess the knowledge that enables them to respond to clues (Hofland & Dardis 1992).

In their study, Kaye et al (1986) demonstrated that patients with chronic symptoms of bulimia generally experience more marked reduction in anxiety than in depression during the course of bingeing and vomiting episodes. They also found that while patterns of bingeing and vomiting appeared to remain stable for each individual, different subjects demonstrated a wide range of mood responses. What is clear from these studies

---

Case study 7.1

Alice is a 22-year-old female single student who has a history of overconcern with her weight and shape, resulting in dietary restraint with episodes of overeating. In July of the year in question she was referred to an eating disorder unit. Alice became concerned about her body weight at the age of 16 and so reduced her food intake. She also reported general feelings of poor self-esteem and low confidence in addition to being preoccupied with her body image. At this time she was not compulsive with exercise and did not abuse laxatives. She did not perceive any particular family problems. Alice's father was retired and overweight but did not appear to have any emotional problems. Her mother was of average weight. Her brother had no particular difficulties. Alice was desperately unhappy after her GCSEs when she moved to a sixth form college. She had left her close friends behind and she felt that she was on the wrong course. For 18 months while she was restricting her food intake, she did not menstruate.

For six months before her referral to the eating disorders unit, Alice was experiencing episodes of binge eating occurring one to two times each week. She would consume large quantities of food that she would normally deny herself (a tub of ice cream and several chocolate bars). Following the binge eating, she would initiate self-induced vomiting and use laxatives. At the time of her referral, she was experiencing 30–40 episodes over a four-week period, usually in the afternoon or late evening.

Alice was entered on to a structured eating programme with four weeks of intervention followed by three follow-up appointments. By October of the same year she felt more positive. She gained weight and she binged only twice and vomited only once. She was asking for help and support from others rather than turning to food. There was a change in her thinking. She wanted to do well at university but also realised that there was more to life than a first class honours degree. By January of the following year, 13 months later, her binging had stopped.

is that bingeing and vomiting do respond to and alter mood states but the mechanisms by which this occurs is still not clear.

A biological relationship between bulimia and depression exists as shown by the fact that when bulimic patients are treated with antidepressants, there is a reduction in binge frequency (Agras et al 1987, Cooper & Fairburn 1986, Gwirtsman et al 1984, Pope & Hudson 1986, Walsh et al 1984). It has also been demonstrated that at normal weight, bulimics show a delayed thyroid stimulating hormone (TSH) response to thyroid releasing hormone (TRH) though the significance of this finding is unclear (Gwirtsman et al 1983).

Anorexia nervosa

Crisp et al (1996) describe anorexia as a disorder that is synchronous with the sense of self (egosyntonic) rather than perceived as alien to self (egodystonic). The egosyntonic state is a situation in which the anorectic takes flight into the anorexia condition where the individual seeks refuge by an unwitting reversal and thereafter avoidance of development (Crisp 1980, Crisp et al 1996). Thus, in anorexia nervosa there is a very deep, unstable biopsychological avoidance stance and a pathological drive to lose weight at all cost, despite the potentially harmful physiological consequences. Distorted body image by the individual coupled with distorted attitudes towards food and eating results in both behaviour and strategies that are adopted to facilitate and disguise weight loss. Indeed it can be argued that since puberty is not under personal control (except through anorexia nervosa) it may be experienced as alien to self or egodystonic. Crisp et al (1996) argue that an essential aspect for healthy development is to experience the impact of puberty as a sense of self or egosyntonic, to own the newly emerging body and feel in charge of it. Sex becomes more important than food in relationships and the link between food, growth and sexuality becomes more apparent.

Robinson & McHugh (1996) have put forward a set of hypotheses about the role of gastric physiology whereby changes in gastric emptying provoke a sensation of fullness or satiation that may encourage or sustain the anorexic behaviour. The same authors add that cholecystokinin (CCK), a brain–gut peptide that is released from the intestines after eating which modulates both food intake and gastric emptying, has a role in anorexia nervosa. CCK inhibits both feeding and gastric emptying and there is evidence from experimental models to suggest that delayed gastric emptying may be an inhibitory factor on food intake in anorexia nervosa. Some studies have shown a higher CCK level in blood of those with anorexia nervosa (Harty et al 1991, Phillipp et al 1991) while others (Geracioti & Liddle 1988, Geracioti et al 1992) found CCK levels to be normal when compared with healthy controls. Kaye et al (1988) observed abnormal serotonin and noradrenaline levels in both low weight and weight-restored anorexic individuals and suggested that not only did these abnormal levels affect appetite, mood, motor activity and metabolism, they also perpetuated the factors in anorexia nervosa. A review by Garner (1993) on the pathogenesis of anorexia nervosa considers both scientific and practice issues and addresses the predisposing, precipitating and perpetuating factors.

Recent studies on cerebral blood oxygenation changes with magnetic resonance imaging (MRI) in a group of female patients (Ellison et al 1998) provide evidence that calorie fear in people who have anorexia nervosa is associated with activation in a limbic and paralimbic network. They suggest that the left amygdala-hippocampal region may mediate conditioned fear to high-calorie foods whereas the insula and anterior cingulate may be involved in autonomic arousal and attentional processes.

Raphael & Lacey (1992) state that genetic, physiological, psychosocial and cultural factors may all play a role in the induction of anorexia nervosa. There is a strong suggestion that a genetic predisposition to anorexia nervosa is indicated as shown by the 50% concordance for anorexia nervosa among the 28 twin pairs compared with 7% concordance in dizygotic twins (Marx 1994). A review by Pieri & Campbell (1999) on several studies done to date seems to support the view that there are several lines of evidence suggesting familial aggregation in anorexia nervosa. Figure 7.3 summarises some of the physiological factors and behav-

---

Case study 7.2

Tracy is a 33-year-old student who had been an inpatient at a regional unit specialising in eating disorders. She had been treated unsuccessfully in other peripheral hospitals in the past for anorexia nervosa. When she was 15 years old, Tracy developed anorexia and by the age of 22 years bulimia was also a feature of her eating disorder. Her periods stopped at the age of 17 years. Her reasons for the eating disorder included self-pressure to perform well at school, concern about her mother, who divorced when Tracy was aged 15 years, being scared of the future and the appearance of a 'new man' in the house.

On admission Tracy weighed 34.3 kg, had a body mass index of 13.5, was anaemic and had parotid gland enlargement due to repeated vomiting (four to five times per day). This is a normal reaction to repeated vomiting. She was taking venlafaxine 75 mg in the morning and 150 mg in the evening and Gaviscon as required for persistent dyspepsia and gastric reflux. She had also been taking iron. Three months following admission her weight had increased to 42.75 kg but a bone scan indicated 25% bone mass loss. She remained anaemic. Throughout her inpatient stay she experienced severe depression and low mood and it was difficult to find the most suitable antidepressant. By six months following her admission, Tracy was more hopeful, needed minimal supervision with her meals and her periods had returned. Her urea and electrolytes were normal, as was her haemoglobin count (12.5), but her zinc was marginally low at 11.6 (μmol/l) (normal range 12.6–20 μmol/l). She continued to gain weight.

> **Case study 7.3**
>
> Richard is a 27-year-old man with a 10-year history of dieting. Richard is a vegan and first dieted when he was 16 years of age. He was first seen in an eating disorders unit seven months ago suffering from anorexia nervosa (anorexia atheletica), diabetes insipidus and osteoporosis of −4 standard deviation. On admission he had a body mass index of 15.2, weighing 43.0 kg (which had reduced from 56 kg to 42.5 kg just before admission), and was exercising for five to six hours a day by brisk walking, running and swimming. Richard was severely restricting his nutritional intake and was drinking copious amounts of fluid. His excessive fluid intake was investigated and found to be due to psychogenic polydipsia and not diabetes insipidus. His urea and electrolytes showed that he had low sodium (127 mmol/l), low creatinine (42 µmol/l) and slightly raised bicarbonate levels (30.7 mmol/l).
>
> Richard had spent six years at boarding school, a period he describes as being very sad, but he did well educationally, managing eight GCSEs, two A-levels and an honours university degree. He alleges that he has an allergy to dairy products, which he avoids. He is happy with soya milk and will tolerate fish. On admission Richard was angry and labile in mood, with lability ranging from tearfulness to elation, and he reported suicidal thoughts and self-harm ideation. Non-verbally his communication pattern showed that he was easily distracted, had poor eye contact and was restless and fidgety. Verbally he was chatty, had an accelerated speech pattern and had flight of ideas. He seemed very anxious when talking about food but denied having a problem with food. Richard was treated with fluoxetine 20 mg daily and a three-stage biopsychosocial intervention programme which enabled him to tackle food difficulties, weight gain, body image intepretation, underlying psychological issues and practical issues related to healthy weight adjustment. Seven months following admission into the eating disorders unit, Richard weighed 59.6 kg, had a positive attitude towards food and was discharged from inpatient care to outpatient care after eight months.

ioural practices seen in anorexia nervosa. The medical complications of anorexia nervosa have been described by other authors (Beumont et al 1993, Fairburn 1993, Puri et al 1996, Sharp & Freeman 1993).

Poor nutrient intake in anorexia nervosa not only leads to low energy levels in the diet and body, but it also results in depletion of glycogen and fat stores, damage to gastrointestinal tract structures, haematological changes and poor homeostatic regulation of body temperature. From a psychosocial behavioural perspective, anorexic individuals isolate themselves socially from family and friends, and when they do not isolate themselves they become irritable and restless in manner and behaviour.

ROLE OF VITAMINS AND MINERALS

Both vitamins and minerals play a significant role as cofactors and coenzymes in the metabolic pathways in general as well as in pathways of several neurotransmitters, especially catecholamines and indoleamines. Deficiencies of vitamins and/or minerals can cause a change in the kinetics of enzymes that are involved in the synthesis or detoxification of substances. For example, the B vitamins involved in intermediary metabolism include thiamine, riboflavin, niacin, pantothenic acid, lipoic acid and biotin (Linder 1991).

Thiamine (B1) deficiency over relatively shorter time spans results in neurasthenia characterised by fatigue, weakness and emotional fatigue, and acute deficiency can cause Wernicke's encephalopathy (Lishman 1998). The issues relating to Wernicke's encephalopathy are discussed later in this chapter.

Westermarck & Antila (1994) discuss several micronutrients whose deficiency is implicated in brain development, neurochemical function, brain metabolism and behaviour. For example with regard to brain development, vitamin B12 deficiency causes hydrocephalus while pyridoxine (B6) deficiency and vitamin E deficiency cause neural tube defects (Scott et al 1990, Westermarck & Antila 1994). The role of pyridoxine in the synthesis and metabolism of the majority of the neurotransmitters and protein hormones such as insulin and growth hormone must not be underestimated.

The characteristics of pyridoxine deficiency disorders include fatigue, nervousness, irritability, depression, insomnia and walking difficulties. In addition dizziness, peripheral neuropathy and neuralgia are also seen (Westermarck & Antila 1994). Depression in women taking oral contraceptives has been linked to deficiency in pyridoxine deficiency since the depression was relieved by pyridoxine replacement in double-blind crossover trials (Adams et al 1973). In some cases pyridoxine deficiency can be induced by certain drugs, such as those that are hydrazine derived, resulting in such symptoms as irritability, peripheral neuropathy and convulsions (Westermarck & Antila 1994). Thiamine deficiency affects both glucose metabolism by interfering with glucose entry into the tricarboxylic acid cycle as well as affecting the synthesis of neurotransmitters glutamic acid and aspartic acid (Westermarck & Antila 1994).

Some macro and micro elements play a significant role in both brain development and functioning. Magnesium deficiency, a condition known as hypomagnesaemia, is characterised by restlessness and psychomotor instability in children, while in adults apathy, anorexia and sometimes hallucinations occur (Westermarck & Antila 1994). Roger (1992) states that it is reasonable to consider magnesium deficiency in chronic fatigue syndrome, depression, panic attacks, Alzheimer's disease and other organic brain syndromes.

ALCOHOL CONSUMPTION AND NUTRITIONAL STATUS

Alcohol is the most commonly used drug in the western world and its abuse significantly affects nutritional status (Auerhahn 1992). In chronic drinkers, alcohol more than often replaces food and apart from its contribution to the total calorific intake, with the exception of wine and beer, it contains limited usable nutrients and its consumption does interfere with the effective utilisation of essential nutrients (Korsten & Lieber 1979, Morgan 1982).

The majority of the problems that result from alcohol abuse are shown in vitamin (especially the B complex group) and mineral deficiencies. Thiamine (vitamin B1) deficiency has been observed in 30–80% of alcoholics (Auerhahn 1992, Morgan 1982, Simpson 1992, Yen 1983) while 50% of pyridoxine deficiency and 35% of niacin deficiency have been reported (Morgan 1982). The factors that lead to thiamine deficiency in alcoholism include substitution of alcohol for vitamin-containing foods, impaired absorption of thiamine from the gastrointestinal tract, poor storage in the liver, reduced phosphorylation to thiamine pyrophosphate and the increased additional requirement for the metabolism of alcohol (Lishman 1998). Chronic alcoholism also leads to a deficiency in folic acid (Halsted 1994). According to Halsted (1990), the aetiology of folate deficiency in chronic alcoholism is multifactorial, as shown by the fact that in acute cases of alcoholism folate availability to bone marrow is decreased, and in chronic cases liver stores of folate are affected due to the 'triple jeopardy' of poor intestinal absorption of folic acid, reduced uptake of folic acid by liver and increased excretion of folic acid by the kidneys. The role of folic acid in mental health has already been discussed in this chapter.

Alcohol abuse may also lead to decreased intake of calcium, iron and phosphorus (Morgan 1982, Lieber 1988), magnesium (Roe 1981) and zinc (Russell 1980). It is believed that zinc has a role in the metabolism and transport of vitamin A to tissues, and combined deficiencies of vitamin A and zinc in many alcoholics have been observed (Auerhahn 1992).

In older adults, the physical and mental effects of alcohol are more pronounced than in the young age groups due to decreased physiological and psychological conditions (Schuckit & Pastor 1979, Simpson 1992, Wattis 1983). Thus, alcohol does interfere with nutritional status through altered absorption, metabolism and excretion of nutrients. A study by Gruchow et al (1985) revealed that alcoholic drinkers had a significantly higher intake of energy than non-drinkers but their intake of non-alcoholic energy decreased as alcohol intake increased. The same authors estimated that between 15% and 41% of alcoholic energy had replaced non-alcoholic energy due to lowered carbohydrate intake.

Since alcohol abusers do not eat a healthy diet, it stands to reason that their micronutrient reserves are also greatly depleted and never or very rarely replenished, thus resulting in nutritional deficiency syndromes of alcohol abuse as summarised by Auerhahn (1992). The neurological disorders that may result from deficiencies related to alcohol abuse include peripheral neuritis, peripheral neuropathy, nutritional amblyopia, cerebellar degeneration and Wernicke-Korsakoff syndrome. In peripheral neuropathy, there is weakness and paraesthesia of lower extremities characterised by diminished deep tendon reflexes in the ankle and by loss of vibratory sense in toes. The presenting features of Wernicke's encephalopathy form a classic triad which includes mental confusion, ataxia (staggering gait) and wavering vision or diplopia on looking to the side (Lishman 1998). Retrospective studies of autopsy-proven cases by Harper et al (1986) showed that this classic triad is not always present. There is a close relationship between Wernicke's encephalopathy and Korsakoff's syndrome as demonstrated by the clear evidence provided by Malamud & Skillicorn (1956) who showed that the location of the cerebral damage is identical in both conditions, the only difference being the acuteness or chronicity of the degree of cerebral damage. Korsakoff's syndrome is often a permanent manifestation of Wernicke's encephalopathy (Lishman 1998). The presenting features in Wernicke-Korsakoff syndrome are ataxia, ophthalmoplegia, confabulation, loss of memory and defective cognitive function (Auerhahn 1992, Korsten & Lieber 1979).

Indeed, while there are benefits in having one or two drinks a day, such as increased longevity (Lopes 1989 cited in Simpson 1992), increased iron storage (Yen 1983), hypnotic effects (Charness et al 1989) and stimulation of appetite (Yen 1983) for moderate drinkers when compared with non-drinkers and heavy drinkers, there is no doubt that excess consumption of alcohol has detrimental effects to physiological and mental functioning.

FOOD SENSITIVITY AND HYPERACTIVITY (CLINICAL ECOLOGY)

The issue of intolerance, allergy and hypersensitivity to food substances by individuals is a complex but interesting one. Some clinicians both in the USA and the UK refer to the area of food sensitivity as clinical ecology. MacDonald (1989) describes food intolerance as an unpleasant reaction to foods that is not psychologically based and the reaction is reproducible under blind conditions, while food allergy is a form of food intolerance in which there is an abnormal immunological reaction.

As early as 1975, Feingold attributed the behaviour seen in some children to commercial additives to foods. Many parents supported this view and reported that their children became restless, irritable and uncontrollable after consuming certain foods or food additives such as dyes, flavours and preservatives (Kinsbourne 1994). However, controlled studies (Harley et al 1978) were unable to demonstrate this conclusively and the satisfactory testing of Feingold's hypothesis has proved to be difficult (Dickerson 1987). Nonetheless this view is still held today by many parents, whatever the scientific world may say. Crook (1975) reports that parents cite cane sugar as one of the triggers of hyperactive behaviour and Bennett & Sherman (1983) recommend the restriction of sugar in hyperactive patients. Other studies of hyperactive children by Prinz et al (1980) found a significant correlation between sugar ingestion and blind ratings of destructive, aggressive or restless behaviour in the playroom but not between sugar ingestion and activity level. In a group of normal children, the opposite pattern of correlation was found. In another study (Behar et al 1984), boys reported to be sugar reactive by their parents were challenged by being asked to consume glucose, sucrose and saccharin, only to produce the opposite effect of decreased motor activity when sugar was given. Kinsbourne (1994) states that the conclusion that can be drawn from these studies is that sugar affects the behaviour of normal children and those with attention deficit hyperactivity disorder in different ways.

David (1987) used tartrazine and benzoic acid in double-blind challenges in children whose parents had reported a definite history of behavioural problems due to these additives and found that none of the children reacted to the additive when challenged. However, Egger et al (1985) demonstrated that the hyperactive children who were more likely to respond to diet therapy were those suffering from atopic symptoms such as eczema or asthma. In another study Pearson et al (1983) confirmed four hypersensitivity reactions to ingested substances out of 23 patients but these same authors found that there was a high incidence of psychiatric disorder in the 19 patients whose belief that they had a food allergy could not be confirmed. These same authors state that on average, there were six complaints out of a total of 16 complaints per patient that included lethargy, head pain of tightness, depression, paraesthesiae, breathlessness, mood swings, irritability, anxiety and panic attacks.

CONCLUSION

The role played by nutrition factors in the mental health of individuals is a crucial one. When one considers the role played by both macro- and micronutrients in growth and development as well as in intermediary metabolism, from the cradle to the grave, it is rather surprising that nutrition issues are not a primary concern of mental health workers. There is enough evidence now to support the view that nutrients have a special role in cognitive functioning and mental homeostasis. In addition to the specific role played by individual nutrients, mealtimes are social occasions that can be used therapeutically by mental health workers to encourage and assess interaction, communication and social skills.

REFERENCES

Adams P W, Wynn V, Rose D P, Folkard J, Strong R 1973 Effect of pyridoxine hydrochloride (vitamin B6) upon depression associated with oral contraception. Lancet 1: 897–904

Agras W S, Dorian B, Kirley B G, Arnow B, Bachman J 1987 Imipramine in the treatment of bulimia: a double-blind controlled study. International Journal of Eating Disorders 6: 29–38

Alpert J E, Fava M 1997 Nutrition and depression: the role of folate. Nutrition Reviews 55(5): 145–149

Alpert M, Silva R, Pouget E (1996) Folate as a predictor of response to sertraline or nortriptylline in geriatric depression. Presented at the 36th annual meeting of NCDEU, Boca Raton, Fl, 28–31 May

Auerhahn C 1992 Recognition and management of alcohol-related nutritional deficiencies. Nurse Practitioner 17(12): 40–49

Barbour B, Szatkowski M, Ingledew N, Attwell D 1989 Arachidonic acid induces a prolonged inhibition of glutamate uptake into glial cells. Nature 342: 918–920

Beck A T, Ward C H, Mendelson M, Mock J, Erbaugh J 1961 An inventory for measuring depression. Archives of General Psychiatry 4: 561–571

Behar D, Rapoport J L, Adams A J, Berg C J, Cornblath M 1984 Sugar challenge testing with children considered behaviourally 'sugar reactive'. Nutrition Behaviour 1: 277–288

Bennett F C, Sherman R 1983 Management of childhood 'hyperactivity' by primary care physicians. Journal of Developmental and Behavioural Paediatrics 4: 88–93

Benton D, Owen D 1993 Is raised blood glucose associated with the relief of tension? Journal of Psychosomatic Research 37(7): 723–735

Benton D, Brett V, Brain P F 1987 Glucose improves attention and reaction to frustration in children. Biological Psychology 24: 95–100

Benton D, Kumari N, Brain B F 1982 Mild hypoglycaemia and questionnaire measures of aggression. Biological Psychology 14: 129–135

Beumont P J V, Russell J D, Touyz S W 1993 Treatment of anorexia nervosa. Lancet 341: 1635–1640

Botez M I, Young S N, Bachevalier J, Gauthier S 1979 Folate deficiency and decreased brain 5–hydroxytryptamine synthesis in man and rat. Nature 278: 182–183

Brobeck J R 1948 Food intake as a mechanism of temperature regulation. Tale Journal of Biological Medicine 20: 545–548

Cannon W B 1898 The movement of the stomach studied by means of the Rontgen Rays. American Journal of Physiology 1: 359

Carlsson M, Carlsson A 1990 Schizophrenia: a subcortical neurotransmitter imbalance syndrome? Schizophrenia Bulletin 16: 425–432

Carney M, Sheffield B F 1970 Associations of subnormal serum folate and vitamin B12 and effects of replacement therapy. Journal of Nervous and Mental Disease 150: 404–412

Carney M W P, Chary T K N, Laundry M et al 1990 Red cell folate concentrations in psychiatric patients. Journal of Affective Disorders 19: 207–213

Chamberlain B, Ervin F R, Pihl R O, Young S N 1987 The effect of raising or lowering tryptophan levels on aggression in vervet monkeys. Pharmacology Biochemistry and Behaviour 28: 503–510

Charness M E, Simon R P, Greenberg D A 1989 Ethanol and the nervous system. New England Journal of Medicine 319: 1318–1330

Christensen O, Christensen E 1988 Fat consumption and schizophrenia. Acta Psychiatrica Scandanavica 78: 587–591

Cooper P J, Fairburn C G 1986 The depressive symptoms of bulimia nervosa. British Journal of Psychiatry 148: 268–274

Coppen A, Chaudry S, Swade C 1986 Folic acid enhances lithium prophylaxis. Journal of Affective Disorder 10: 9–10

Crisp A H 1980 Anorexia nervosa: let me be. Academic Press, London

Crisp A H, Joughin N, Halek C, Bowyer C 1996 Anorexia nervosa: the wish to change – self-help and discovery: the thirty steps, 2nd edn. Psychology Press, Hove

Crook W G 1975 Food allergy – the great masquerader. Paediatric Clinics of North America 22: 227–238

David T 1987 Reactions to dietary tartrazine. Archives of Disease in Childhood 62(2): 119–122

Dickerson J W T 1987 The hyperactive child: dietary management? Professional Nurse 3(3): 92–95

Di Pietro L, Anda R F, Williamson D F, Stunkard A J 1992 Depressive symptoms and weight change in a national cohort of adults. International Journal of Obesity and Related Metabolic Disorders 16(10): 745–753

Dippel N M, Becknal B K 1987 Bulimia. Journal of Psychosocial Nursing 25(9): 13–17

Egger J, Carter C M, Graham P J, Cumley D, Soothill J F 1985 Controlled trial of oligoantigenic diet in the treatment of hyperlunetic syndrome. Lancet 1: 540–544

Ellison Z, Foong J, Howard R, Bullmore E, Williams S, Treasure J 1998 Functional anatomy of calorie fear in anorexia nervosa (letter). Lancet 352 (9135): 1192

Fairburn C G 1993 Eating disorders. In: Kendell R E, Zealley A K (eds) Companion to psychiatric studies, 5th edn. Churchill Livingstone, Edinburgh, p 525–541

Fava M, Borus J S, Alpert J E, Nierenberg A A, Rosenbaum J F, Bottiglieri T 1997 Folate, B12 and homocysteine in major depressive disorder. American Journal of Psychiatry 154: 426–428

Feingold B F 1975 Hyperkinesis and learning disabilities linked to artificial food flavours and colours. American Journal of Nursing 75: 797–803

Fernstrom J D, Wurtman J R 1971 Brain serotonin content increase following ingestion of carbohydrate. Science 174: 1023–1025

Fernstrom J D, Wurtman J R 1972 Brain serotonin content; physiological regulation by plasma neutral amino acids. Science 178: 414–416

Garner D M 1993 Pathogenesis of anorexia nervosa. Lancet 341: 1631–1635

Geracioti T, Liddle R 1988 Impaired cholecystokinin secretion in bulimia nervosa. New England Journal of Medicine 319: 683–688

Geracioti T D, Liddle R A, Altemus M, Demitrack M A, Gold P W 1992 Regulation of appetite and cholecystokinin secretion in anorexia nervosa. American Journal of Psychiatry 149: 958–961

Ghadirian A M, Ananth J, Engelsmann F 1980 Folic acid deficiency and depression. Psychosomatics 21(11): 926–929

Godfrey P S A, Toone B K, Carney M W P et al 1990 Enhancement of recovery from psychiatric illness by methylfolate. Lancet 336: 392–395

Gruchow H W, Sobocinski K A, Barboriak J J, Scheller J G 1985 Alcohol consumption, nutrient intake and relative body weight among US adults. American Journal of Clinical Nutrition 42: 289–295

Gwirtsman H E, Kaye W, Weintraub M, Jimerson D C 1984 Pharmacologic treatment of eating disorders. Psychiatric Clinics of North America 7: 863–878

Gwirtsman H E, Roy-Byrne P, Yager J, Gerner R H 1983 Neuroendocrine abnormalities in bulimia. American Journal of Psychiatry 140(5): 559–563

Halsted C H 1990 Intestinal absorption of dietary folates. In: Piciano M F, Stokstad E L R, Gregory J F (eds) Folic acid metabolism in health and disease. Contemporary issues in clinical nutritrion. Alan R Liss, New York, p 23–45

Halsted C H 1994 Water soluble vitamins. In: Garrow J S, James W P T (eds) Human nutrition and dietetics. Churchill Livingstone, Edinburgh, p 239–263

Hamilton M 1960 A ratings scale for depression. Journal of Neurology and Neurosurgical Psychiatry 23: 56–62

Hardy R H 1984 Endocrine physiology. Edward Arnold, London

Harley J P, Ray R S, Tomasi L et al 1978 Hyperkinesis and food additives: testing the Feingold hypothesis. Paediatrics 61: 818–828

Harper A E, Benevenga M J, Wohleuter R H 1970 Effects of ingestion of disproportionate amounts of amino acids. Physiological reviews 50: 428–558

Harper C G, Giles M, Finlay-Jones R 1986 Clinical signs in the Wernicke-Korsakoff complex: a retrospective analysis of 131 cases diagnosed at necropsy. Journal of Neurology, Neurosurgery and Psychiatry 49: 341–345

Harty R F, Pearson P H, Solomon T E, McGuigan J E 1991 Cholecystokinin, vasoactive intestinal peptide and peptide histidine methionine responses to feeding in anorexia nervosa. Regulatory Peptides 36: 141–150

Herbert V 1961 Experimental nutritional folate deficiency in man. Transactions of the Association of American Physicians 75: 307–320

Hofland S L, Dardis P O 1992 Bulimia nervosa. Associated physical problems. Journal of Psychosocial Nursing & Mental Health Services 30(2): 23–27

Holmes S 1986 Determinants of food intake. Nursing 7: 260–264

Hunter R, Jones M, Jones T, Matthews D 1967 Serum B12 and folate concentrations in mental patients. British Journal of Psychiatry 113: 1291–1295

Jimerson D C, Lesem M D, Kaye W H, Brewerton T D 1992 Low serotonin and dopamine metabolite concentrations in cerebrospinal fluid from bulimic patients with frequent binge episodes. Archives of General Psychiatry 49: 132–138

Kaye W H, Ebert M H, Lake C R 1988 Disturbances in brain neurotransmitter systems in anorexia nervosa: a review of CSF studies. In: B J Blinder, B F Chaitin, R S Goldstein (eds) The eating disorders. PMA, New York, p 215–225

Kaye W H, Ebert M H, Gwirtsman H E, Weiss S R 1984 Differences in brain serotonergic metabolism between nonbulimic and bulimic patients with anorexia nervosa American Journal of Psychiatry 141: 1598–1601

Kaye W H, Gwirtsman H E, George D T, Weiss S R, Jimerson D C 1986 Relationship of mood alterations to bingeing behaviour in bulimia. British Journal of Psychiatry 149: 479–485

Kaye W H, Ballanger J C, Lydiard B et al 1990 CSF monoamine levels in normal-weight bulimia: evidence for abnormal noradrenergic activity. American Journal of Psychiatry 147: 225–229

Kennedy G C 1953 Role of depot fat in hypothalamic control of food intake. Proceedings of the Royal Society 140(B): 578–592

Kinsbourne M 1994 Sugar and the hyperactive child (editorial). New England Journal of Medicine 330(5): 355–356

Korsten M A, Lieber C S 1979 Nutrition in alcoholics. Medical Clinics of North America 63(5): 963–970

Levin P A, Falko J M, Dixon K, Gallup E M, Saunders W 1980 Benign parotid enlargement in bulimia. Annals of Internal Medicine 93: 827–829

Lieber C S 1988 The influence of alcohol on nutritional status. Nutrition Reviews 46(7): 241–254

Linder M C 1991 Nutrition and metabolism of vitamins. In: Linder M C (ed) Nutritional biochemistry and metabolism with clinical applications, 2nd edn. Prentice-Hall, London, p 111–189

Lishman W A 1998 Organic psychiatry – the psychological consequences of cerebral disorder, 3rd edn. Blackwell Science, Oxford

Lopes M M 1989 [Alcohol and the heart]. Revista Portuguesa de Cardiologia 8: 435–439

MacDonald A 1989 Food allergy and intolerance. Paediatric Nursing 1(5): 14–16

Malamud N, Skillicorn S A 1956 Relationship between the Wernicke and the Korsakoff syndrome. Archives of Neurology and Psychiatry 76: 585–596

Marx R D 1994 Anorexia nervosa: theories of etiology. In: Alexander-Mott L A, Lumsden D B (eds) Understanding eating disorders. Taylor & Francis, London, p 123–134

Mayer J 1953 Glucostatic mechanism of regulation of food intake. New England Journal of Medicine 249(1): 13–16

Mayer J, Bates M W 1951 mechanism of regulation of food intake. Federation Proceedings 10: 389

Mayer J, Bates M W, Van Itallie T B 1952 Blood sugar and food intake in rats with lesions of anterior hypothalamus. Metabolism 1: 340–348

Meades S 1993 Suggested community psychiatric nursing interventions with clients suffering from anorexia nervosa and bulimia nervosa. Journal of Advanced Nursing 18: 364–390

Mellor J E, Laugharne J D E, Peet M 1996 Omega-3 fatty acid supplementation in schizophrenic patients. Human Psychopharmacology 11: 39–46

Morgan M Y 1982 Alcohol and nutrition. British Medical Bulletin 38(1): 21–29

Odegard O 1956 The incidence of psychosis in various occupations. International Journal of Social Psychiatry 2: 85–104

Pearson D J, Rix K J B, Bentley S J 1983 Food allergy: how much in the mind? A clinical and psychiatric study of suspected food hypersensitivity. Lancet 4: 1259–1261

Peet M, Laugharne J D E, Horrobin D F, Reynolds G P 1994 Arachidonic acid: a common link in the biology of schizophrenia. Archives of General Psychiatry 51: 665–666

Phillipp E, Pirke K, Kellner M, Krieg J 1991 Disturbed cholecystokinin secretion in patients with eating disorders. Life Sciences 48: 2443–2450

Pieri L F, Campbell D A 1999 Understanding the genetic predisposition to anorexia nervosa. European Eating Disorders Review 7: 1–12

Pope H G, Hudson J I 1986 Antidepressant drug therapy for bulimia: current status. Journal of Clinical Psychiatry 47: 339–345

Prinz R J, Roberts W A, Hantman E 1980 Dietary collerates of hyperactive behaviour in children. Journal of Consultative Clinical psychology 48: 760–769

Puri B K, Laking P J, Treasaden I H 1996 Textbook of psychiatry. Churchill Livingstone, Edinburgh, p 331–343

Ramchand C N, Ramchand R, Hemmings G P 1992 RBC and serum folate concentrations in neuroleptic-treated and neuroleptic-free schizophrenic patients. Journal of Nutritional Medicine 3: 303–309

Raphael F J, Lacey J H 1992 Sociocultural aspects of eating disorders. Annals of Medicine 24: 293–296

Reynolds E H 1967 Effects of folic on the mental state and fit-frequency of drug-treated epileptic patients. Lancet 1: 1086–1088

Reynolds E H 1979 Cerebrospinal fluid folate: clinical studies. In: Botez M I, Reynolds E H (eds) Folic acid in neurology, psychiatry and internal medicine. Raven Press, New York, p 195–303

Reynolds E H, Preece J M, Bailey J, Coppen A 1970 Folate deficiency in depressive illness. British Journal of Psychiatry 117: 287–292

Robinson P H, McHugh P R 1996 A physiology of starvation that sustains eating disorders. In: Szmukler G, Dare C, Treasure J (eds) Handbook of eating disorders: theory, treatment and research. Wiley, Chichester, p 109–123

Roe D A 1981 Nutritional concerns in the alcoholic. Journal of the American Dietetic Association 78: 17–20

Roger S 1992 Chemical sensitivity: breaking the paralysing paradigm: how knowledge of chemical sensitivity enhances the treatment of chronic disease. Internal Medicine World Report 7: 13–41

Royston M C, Lewis S W 1993 Brain pathology in schizophrenia: development or degenerative? Current Opinion in Psychiatry 6: 70–73

Russell R M 1980 Vitamin A and zinc metabolism in alcoholism. American Journal of Clinical Nutrition 33(12): 2741–2749.

Sartorius N, Jablensky A, Shapiro R 1978 Cross-cultural differences in the short-term prognosis of schizophrenic psychoses. Schizophrenia Bulletin 4: 102–113

Schuckit M A, Pastor P A 1979 Alcohol-related pschopathology in the aged. In: Kaplan O J (ed) Psychopathology of aging. Academic Press, New York, p 211–224

Scott J M, Kirke P N, Weir D G 1990 The role of nutrition in neural tube defects. Annual Review of Nutrition 10: 277–295

Sharp C W, Freeman C P L 1993 The medical complications of anorexia nervosa. British Journal of Psychiatry 162: 452–462

Simpson P M 1992 Alcohol consumption in the elderly. Nutrition Research Reviews 5: 153–166

Spector R 1979 Cerebrospinal fluid folate and the blood–brain barrier. In: Botez M I, Reynolds E H (eds) Folic acid in neurology, psychiatry and internal medicine. Raven Press, New York, p 187–194

Spring B, Chiodo D J 1987 Carbohydrates, tryptophan and behaviour: a methodological review. Psychological Bulletin 102: 234–256

Stunkard A, Fernstrom M H, Price A, Frank E, Kupfer D J 1990 Direction of weight change in recurrent depression. Archives of General Psychiatry 47: 860

Sullivan M, Karlson J, Sjostrom L et al 1993 Swedish obese subjects (SOS) an intervention study of obesity. Baseline evaluation of health and psychosocial functioning in the first 1743 subjects examined. International Journal of Obesity and Related Metabolic Disorders 17(9): 503–512

Sundby P, Nyhus P 1963 Major and minor psychiatric disorders in males in Oslo. Acta Psychiatrica Scandanavica 39: 519–547

Thayer R E 1987 Energy, tiredness, and tension effects of a sugar snack versus moderate exercise. Journal of Personality and Social Psychology 52(1): 119–125

Walsh B T, Stewart J W, Roose S P, Gladis M, Glassman A H 1984 Treatment of bulimia with phenelzine: a double-blind, placebo-controlled study. Archives of General Psychiatry 41: 1105–1109

Wattis J P 1983 Alcohol and old people. British Journal of Psychiatry 143: 306–307

Weltzin T E, Fernstrom M H, Kaye W H 1994 Serotonin and bulimia nervosa. Nutrition Reviews 52(12): 399–408

Westermarck T, Antila E 1994 Diet in relation to the nervous system. In: Garrow J S, James W P T (eds) Human nutrition and dietetics, 9th edn. Churchill Livingstone, Edinburgh, p 651–667

World Health Organization 1979 Schizophrenia: an international follow-up study. Wiley, New York

Yen P K 1983 Alcohol – the drug that's also a nutrient. Geriatric Nursing 4(6): 390, 397

Young S N, Smith S E, Pihl R O, Ervin F R 1985 Tryptophan depletion causes a rapid lowering of mood in normal males. Psychopharmacology 87: 173–177

Zung W W, Coppedge H M, Green R L 1974 The evaluation of depressive symptomatology: a triadic approach. Psychotherapy and Psychosomatics 24(2): 170–174

8

Psychopharmacology

Key Points

- The monoamine theory of affective disorders does not fully explain the disorder of synaptic transmission or the action of psychopharmacological agents
- Receptor adaptation is important in the long-term action of psychotropic drugs
- Mental health nurses have a professional responsibility to keep up to date with existing and new drugs used in the treatment of mental health problems

Psychopharmacology refers to the use and study of drugs that act on the central nervous system and modify mood, thought, perception and behaviour. Despite concerns over the use of drugs, their therapeutic use remains a fundamental part of the management of some individuals with mental health problems. Mental health nurses still have a major responsibility to administer prescribed drugs safely and appropriately, to educate and empower individuals who are receiving prescribed drugs, and to observe for and act appropriately with regard to drug side-effects. It is important therefore that mental health professionals should have some understanding of the different groups of drugs used in the management of individuals with mental health problems. Much of that knowledge will be updated in the clinical setting, therefore the purpose of this chapter is to provide the relevant background.

Over the past four decades, as a result of major advances in psychopharmacology, the classification of drugs used has been expanded and modified. Table 8.1 provides a list of the major drug groups. All except hypnotics are considered in this chapter; hypnotics are discussed in Chapter 9.

Table 8.1 Classification of psychopharmacological drugs

Type	Drug group (selected)	Example
Antipsychotics	Phenothiazines	Chlorpromazine
	Thioxanthenes	Flupenthixol
	Dibenzapines	Clozapine
	Butyrophenones	Haloperidol
	Diphenylbutylpiperidines	Pimozide
Antidepressants	Tricyclic and related	Amitriptyline
		Lofepramine
		Trazodone
	Selective serotonin reuptake inhibitors and related	Fluoxetine
		Paroxetine
		Venlafaxine
		Nefazodone
	Monoamine oxidase inhibitors	Phenelzine
		Tranylcypromine
	Reversible inhibitors of monoamine oxidase A (RIMAs)	Moclobemide
Mood stabilisers	Lithium	Lithium carbonate/citrate
		Carbamazipine
Anxiolytics	Benzodiazepines	Alprazolam
		Chlordiazepoxide
		Diazepam
	Azapirones	Buspirone
Hypnotics	Benzodiazepines	Flurazepam
		Loprazolam
		Temazepam
	Cyclopyrrolones	Zopiclone
	Imidazopyrimidines	Zolpidem

HOW DO PSYCHOTROPIC DRUGS ALTER BRAIN ACTIVITY?

As identified in earlier chapters, the neurotransmitters acetylcholine, noradrenaline, dopamine, serotonin (5HT) and GABA are implicated in the development of mental health problems. Attention has therefore been directed at studying the way the release and action of these neurotransmitters at the synapse are modified by psychotropic drugs.

A number of mechanisms have been identified by which psychotropic drugs alter synaptic activity (Leonard 1997). To simplify matters and consistent with the activity of the major psychotropic drugs commonly used, psychotropic drugs may produce an effect by:

- modifying the reuptake of a neurotransmitter into the presynaptic neurone
- activating or inhibiting postsynaptic receptors
- inhibition of enzyme activity.

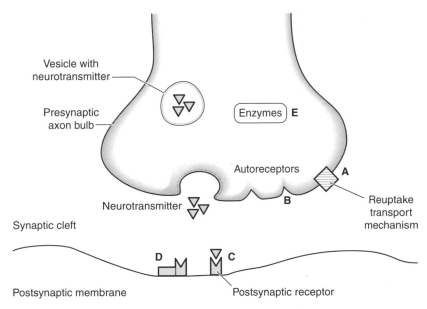

Figure 8.1 The major mechanisms of action for psychotropic drugs.
(A) Reuptake of the neurotransmitter can be blocked (e.g. SSRIs, tricyclic antidepressants). (B) Autoreceptors may be blocked thus increasing the release of neurotransmitters (e.g. some antidepressants). (C) Postsynaptic receptors may be blocked (e.g. neuroleptics). (D) Postsynaptic receptor complexes may be stimulated (e.g. benzodiazepines). (E) Enzymes that inactivate the neurotransmitter may be inhibited (e.g. MAOIs).

Figure 8.1 provides a summary of the major ways in which specific drugs are thought to exert their effects.

A general mechanism that seems to be of importance with regard to the long-term effects of psychotropic drugs on synaptic activity involves *receptor adaptation* (Leonard 1997). Clinical experience supports the view that psychotropic drugs, while profoundly altering neurotransmission and synaptic activity after a single dose, do not produce symptomatic improvement until after two to three weeks. This has led to the proposal that psychotropic drugs work by producing subtle changes in receptor function that occur as a secondary effect of the biochemical change (Leonard 1997).

DRUGS USED IN THE TREATMENT OF DEPRESSION

There is general agreement that the concentrations of the neurotransmitters noradrenaline, dopamine and 5HT within the synapse (and therefore their effects) are reduced by the high-affinity, energy-dependent mechanisms whereby the neurotransmitters are transported into the presynaptic neurone (reuptake). The logical progression of this is to develop drugs that can inhibit the reuptake of these neurotransmitters and hence prolong their concentration within the synapse.

Tricyclic antidepressants (TCAs)

TCAs have been the most important group of antidepressants used in clinical practice. However, the need for a group of drugs that act more quickly and have fewer side-effects has led to the development of newer atypical drugs. Tricyclic antidepressants, including, for example, imipramine, amitriptyline, lofepramine and the newer related drugs maprotiline and mianserin, are potent inhibitors of noradrenaline and/or 5HT reuptake.

Mechanism of pharmacological action

The main effect of TCAs is to block the uptake of amines at nerve endings, probably by competing for the membrane-bound protein carrier that forms part of the reuptake transport system. Most TCAs inhibit noradrenaline and 5HT uptake, with much less effect on dopamine transport. In the conventional TCAs there appears to be little selectivity between blocking the uptake of one amine compared to another but when looking at the group as a whole, TCAs do seem to have a broad spectrum of action (Table 8.2). Importantly, TCAs also act on other neurotransmitter receptors, particularly muscarinic cholinergic receptors, histamine receptors and 5HT receptors.

Table 8.2 Pharmacological action of some tricyclic and related antidepressant agents

Drug	Inhibition of uptake			Affinties for receptor	
	5HT	NA	DA	Muscarinic anticholinergic	Antihistamine
Amitriptyline	++	+++	±	+++	+++
Clomipramine	+++	+	−	++	±
Imipramine	++	+	±	+	+
Paroxetine	+++	−	−	±	−
Fluoxetine	+++	−	−	−	−
Lofepramine	−	++	−	+	?
Citalopram	+++	−	−	−	−
Fluvoxamine	+++	−	−	−	−
Venlafaxine	++	++	±	−	−
Nefazodone	++	++	−	−	−
Maproteline	−	+++	±	±	+
Mianserin	−	+	+	−	++

Modified from Trimble M R 1996 Biological psychiatry, 2nd edn. Copyright John Wiley & Sons Limited. Reproduced with permission.

Clomipramine seems to have stronger effects on 5HT reuptake than on noradrenaline compared to amitriptyline and it has fewer anticholinergic effects. Indeed amitriptyline seems to have a greater effect on nor-adrenaline transport than on 5HT (Leonard 1997, Trimble 1996). Of the tricyclic related group of antidepressants, maprotiline, a tetracyclic, is a noradrenaline reuptake inhibitor with fewer anticholinergic effects. However, it is associated with an increased risk of seizures and is there-fore contraindicated when there is a history of epilepsy. Trazadone has an efficacy similar to that of TCAs but has no anticholinergic properties and is largely free of cardiovascular side-effects. It acts as a 5HT reuptake inhibitor and blocks α_2-adrenoceptors on the presynaptic neurone thus increasing the release of noradrenaline into the synapse.

Unwanted effects

The unwanted side-effects of TCAs (Table 8.3) are usually minor and transient but they may on occasions prove to be so troublesome that they have an impact on compliance and may lead to absolute failure to com-ply. In addition, some drugs, for example amitriptyline, are particularly dangerous in overdosage.

Generally tricyclic and related (atypical) antidepressants are divided according to the extent to which they produce sedation. Amitriptyline, clomipramine, dothiepin, maprotiline and trimipramine, for example, have greater sedative properties than imipramine, lofepramine, nortripty-line and viloxazine. As would be expected, individuals with agitation superimposed on the depression may benefit from the drugs with greater sedative properties.

As already stated, anticholinergic effects are a feature of tricyclic and related antidepressants. Broadly, anticholinergic effects include drowsi-ness, dry mouth, blurred vision, constipation and urinary retention. Some tolerance to these side-effects does seem to develop over time. Postural hypotension has been reported in all age groups. Occasionally, arrhythmias and heart block do seem to develop following the use of this group of antidepressants and this is a consideration when judging the possible issue of self-harm as they are highly dangerous in overdosage. Convulsions have been associated with maprotiline and hepatic and haematological reactions with mianserin. TCAs potentiate the effects of alcohol, and respiratory depression may occur following heavy drinking (Rang et al 1995).

It is recommended that monoamine oxidase inhibitors (MAOIs) should not be started until at least one week after a tricyclic or related antidepressant drug has been stopped. Conversely, tricyclic or related antidepressant drugs should not be commenced within two weeks of stopping an MAOI.

Table 8.3 The main unwanted effects of selected antidepressant agents

Antidepressant	Unwanted effects

Tricyclic antidepressants	Sedation
	Antimuscarinic: dry mouth
	          constipation
	          blurred vision
	          retention of urine
	Postural hypotension
	Cardiac arrhythmias and heart block
	Seizures

Tricyclic related	As for TCA but fewer antimuscarinic effects Increased risk of seizures (maproteline) Haematological disturbance (mianserin)
SSRIs	Nausea Diarrhoea Anxiety and restlessness Insomnia Headache
MAOI	Postural hypotension Weight gain Insomnia Headache Constipation Agitation and tremor Interaction with tyramine
RIMAs	Insomnia Dizziness Nausea Headache Restlessness Agitation

Selective serotonin reuptake inhibitors (SSRIs) and related antidepressants

The first of this type of antidepressant, zimeldine, proved to be neurotoxic. Several SSRIs are now available and they seem to be effective antidepressants with a good safety profile. While they may be in the same group they have a wide variety of pharmacokinetic and pharmacodynamic properties. The main SSRIs used in current clinical practice are:

- citalopram (Cipramil)
- fluoxetine (Prozac)
- fluvoxamine (Faverin)
- paroxetine (Seroxat)
- sertraline (Lustral).

All of them selectively inhibit the reuptake of 5HT, but fluoxetine is the least potent for the inhibition of 5HT reuptake. Inhibition of the 5HT presynaptic transporter occurs within hours, with recovery to the activity of serotonin neurones occurring over 14 days (Montigny & Blier 1985).

Unwanted effects

While the overall efficacy of the SSRIs does not seem to differ significantly from that of the standard TCAs, the side-effect and toxicity profiles do differ (Table 8.3). The main advantages of the SSRIs are the lack of cardiac side-effects, weight gain and sedation, commonly associated with the traditional TCAs. The commonest side-effects, which are dose related, are gastrointestinal in nature. Nausea is usually transient but occasionally may persist and affect compliance. Loss of appetite seems to be more pronounced in overweight individuals. Central nervous system (CNS) side-effects, including insomnia, restlessness and anxiety are common but usually relatively minor. Headaches and tremors may also occur. Hypersensitivity reactions including angioedema, pruritus and urticaria have been reported. Sexual dysfunction, with delayed ejaculation and anorgasmia, is another side-effect of SSRIs and related antidepressant drugs. There have been reports of increased violence and occasionally aggression in individuals treated with fluoxetine and reports of an increase in suicide rate. However, reports of such effects were largely restricted to the USA, the debate has largely subsided and the association has not been established through systematic randomised controlled trials (Rang et al 1995, Bond & Lader 1996).

SSRIs should not be stopped abruptly but gradually discontinued by dose tapering or alternate day administration. In particular, withdrawal syndrome, which includes dizziness, paraesthesia, anxiety, sleep disturbance, agitation, tremor, nausea, sweating and confusion, has been associated with the abrupt discontinuation of paroxetine.

The combination of SSRIs with MAOIs is potentially very dangerous as it can result in 'serotonin syndrome' associated with tremor, hyperthermia and cardiovascular collapse (Rang et al 1995). An SSRI or related antidepressant should not be started within two weeks of stopping an MAOI. Due to the long half-life associated with SSRIs, MAOIs should not be started until after two weeks in the case of paroxetine and sertraline and after five weeks for fluoxetine.

Venlafaxine, nefazodone and reboxetine have been introduced as antidepressants. Venlafaxine is thought to inhibit the reuptake of serotonin and noradrenaline, while nefazodone inhibits the reuptake of serotonin and also selectively blocks $5HT_2$ receptors. Both are related to SSRIs. Reboxetine is a selective reuptake inhibitor of noradrenaline.

Monoamine oxidase inhibitors (MAOIs)

MAOIs were first introduced to treat tuberculosis but were found to have mood-elevating effects. Due to the potential serious side-effects of traditional MAOIs, their use has largely been superseded by TCAs and SSRIs. However, with the emergence of reversible MAOIs, interest in the use of this group of antidepressants has been raised.

As outlined in previous chapters, monoamine oxidase (MAO) is found in nearly all tissues and exists in two similar but distinct molecular forms, named A and B (Benedetti & Dostert 1992). Monoamine oxidase A (MAOA) acts on the substrates noradrenaline and serotonin whereas monoamine oxidase B (MAOB) acts on phenylethylamine. Tyramine and dopamine are substrates for both. The inhibition of MAO using irreversible and reversible MAOIs leads to the widespread accumulation of amines (5HT, noradrenaline and dopamine). Of the irreversible MAOIs, phenelzine and isocarboxazid are the drugs of choice as they have less stimulant action compared to tranylcypromine. Moclobemide acts by reversible inhibition of MAOA and is often termed a RIMA (reversible inhibitor of MAOA).

Clinically MAOIs seem to offer little in the treatment of general depression when compared to TCAs and SSRIs. However, there appears to be some evidence that they have a place in the treatment of individuals with 'atypical depression' (Trimble 1996). Although not clearly defined, atypical depression includes depression with associated features of hypochondriasis, somatic anxiety, social phobias, agoraphobia, panic attacks and hysteria. Response to MAOIs may not be observed until three weeks after the initial administration. Indeed an increase in the dose prescribed may be required after one to two weeks depending upon the response of the individual. As with TCAs the mechanism for the antidepressant effect of MAOIs is not fully understood and the delayed clinical response may suggest similar neuronal receptor adaptive changes as those found with long-term TCA therapy.

Unwanted effects

Adverse effects commonly associated with irreversible MAOIs include postural hypotension and dizziness. In addition, autonomic side-effects may occur including dry mouth and skin, sexual dysfunction, constipation and blurred vision. Localised peripheral oedema, which may be unilateral, may occur as an unusual side-effect. Acute psychotic episodes with hypomanic behaviour and hallucinations may occur in individuals who are predisposed to the development of schizophrenia.

The major concern with the use of MAOIs is the interaction which can occur with specific foods and other amine drugs, such as those found in many cough and decongestant preparations. MAOIs inhibit the enzymatic breakdown of amines leading to an accumulation of amine neurotransmitters (e.g. noradrenaline). The result is that MAOIs can potentiate the cardiovascular effects and in particular the pressor effects of amine neurotransmitters. This may result in an excessive and dangerous elevation in blood pressure.

The 'cheese reaction' is a phenomenon resulting from irreversible MAO inhibition when normal amounts of the amino acid tyramine are ingested. Tyramine is an indirectly acting sympathomimetic amine and at the neurone ending it displaces noradrenaline from the presynaptic vesicles into the cytoplasm. From there noradrenaline either leaks out into the synapse to produce a response or is degraded by MAO. Tyramine is normally metabolised by MAO present in the wall of the gastrointestinal tract and in the liver, so little dietary tyramine enters the systemic circulation. Due to the action of irreversible MAOIs, tyramine reaches the systemic circulation and increased amounts of noradrenaline leave the nerve ending, producing an enhanced pressor effect. The earliest warning sign of the cheese effect is the development of an acute throbbing headache as a consequence of severe elevation of the blood pressure. Mental health nurses and other health professionals need to provide effective nutritional advice and education for individuals prescribed irreversible MAOIs.

Moclobemide (RIMA) is claimed to produce less potentiation of the pressor effect of dietary tyramine, although individuals still should be advised to avoid eating large amounts of tyramine-rich food (Box 8.1) and to avoid cough mixtures that contain sympathomimetic drugs such as ephedrine, pseudoephedrine and phenylpropanolamine.

Box 8.1   Foods to avoid when taking MAOIs

Cheese: especially matured (excludes cottage cheese or cream cheese)
Marmite, Bovril and other protein extracts
Pickled herring, liver, game, whole broad beans
Yoghurt
Alcoholic drinks: especially chianti and red wine (excludes spirits)

ANTIDEPRESSANTS AND CLINICAL EFFECTIVENESS: THE MECHANISM?

It is important to state that the original monoamine theory of depression, in which it is suggested that antidepressants work simply by enhancing monoamine neurotransmission, is no longer tenable. It is well recognised that despite immediate changes in the concentrations of neurotransmitters, the clinical effects of antidepressants are not observed until two to three weeks after the initial start of the drug treatment. This phenomenon does not fit easily with the monoamine hypothesis of depression. Attempts have been made to explain this both pharmacologically and biochemically, and more recently attention has been given to the long-term effects of antidepressant agents on the sensitivity of catecholamine receptors and in particular the downregulation of β-adrenoceptor activity (Trimble 1996).

Long-term administration of antidepressants has been found to lead to both the reduced number of binding sites and a reduction in the functional response of β- and α_2-adrenoceptors (Sulser 1984) and $5HT_2$ receptors (Rang et al 1995). The reduction in the sensitivity of receptors and in the number of receptor binding sites is called *downregulation*. Impaired presynaptic inhibition by the downregulation of α_2-adrenoceptors, resulting in increased noradrenergic impulse flow and turnover, may explain the clinical improvement. However, loss of β-adrenoceptors does not fit comfortably with the monoamine hypothesis as β-adrenoceptor blockers do not act as antidepressants. Indeed some of the newer antidepressants, for example mianserin, paroxetine and fluoxetine, fail to downregulate β-adrenoceptors, suggesting that this change is not in itself sufficient to explain the effects of antidepressants as a whole (Trimble 1996).

The downregulation of adrenoceptor activity seems to be dependent upon an intact presynaptic serotonergic neuronal input. Indeed the introduction of SSRI antidepressants has focused the attention on to 5HT and 5HT receptors. As already addressed in this book, a number of 5HT receptor subtypes are found within the CNS. Modulation of the postsynaptic $5HT_2$ receptor and the presynaptic $5HT_{1A}$ autoreceptor has been implicated in the genesis of depression and in the clinical effects of antidepressants. It is suggested that there may be supersensitivity of the postsynaptic $5HT_2$ receptor which leads to decreased function of $5HT_{1A}$. The presynaptic $5HT_{1A}$ receptor normally autoregulates the release of serotonin from the presynaptic neurone. However, the interaction between and the relative contribution of each receptor is not yet fully understood.

Trimble (1996) suggests that SSRIs initially lead to an excess amount of 5HT flooding the synapse, resulting in a 'shutting down' of the system. Then, over a period of time, consistent with the delayed clinical action of antidepressant drugs, there is resumption of activity but with a further decrease in the sensitivity of $5HT_{1A}$. This subsensitivity of $5HT_{1A}$ enhances serotonin release and leads to normalisation of $5HT_2$ receptor function. Depression may be more related to upregulation of postsynaptic receptor sites which could be related to decreased intrasynaptic levels of neurotransmitters due to hypersensitivity of presynaptic receptors.

DRUGS USED IN THE TREATMENT OF MANIA AND BIPOLAR DISORDERS

Biochemical basis of mania

While the biochemical basis of mania is not fully understood, the monoamine theory associated with depression has been applied to the understanding of mania. Simplistically, the monoamine theory explains the development of mania as being due to a relative excess of noradrenaline and possibly dopamine within the central synapses. There may also be an associated deficit in the availability of acetylcholine and serotonin (Leonard 1997). However, this hypothesis is based on a limited number of studies.

Some attention has been given to the influence of serotonin. Mania has been reported in patients who have been treated with tryptophan and clomipramine (Leonard 1997). Unlike in depression where 5HT uptake into platelets is reduced, in mania 5HT uptake seems to be increased before treatment, but following treatment this normalises (Leonard 1997).

Lithium salts

The psychotropic nature of lithium was discovered by the Australian psychiatrist Cade in 1949 (Rang et al 1995). Lithium is a metallic cation which is found widespread in soil and nature and it forms complex mineral salts. Lithium salts are indicated for the prophylactic treatment of mania and bipolar mood swings and have a place in the prophylaxis of unipolar depression.

Mode of action

Despite the relative chemical simplicity of lithium salts, the mode of action of this group of drugs is both complex and only partially understood. Lithium mimics the effects of sodium and interacts with a number of other cations in cellular processes, for example sodium, potassium, calcium and magnesium. Lithium does seem to reduce the sodium content of the brain, and increases central serotonin synthesis and noradrenaline reuptake in the brain (Leonard 1997, Trimble 1996). In excitable tissues lithium permeates the fast sodium ion channels but unlike sodium it is not pumped out of the cell as quickly, so accumulation of lithium inside the cell occurs. This leads to a partial loss of intracellular potassium and partial depolarisation of the neurone (Rang et al 1995).

The mechanisms responsible for the main therapeutic effects of lithium involve changes to the second messenger systems located in the cell. These second messenger systems are required to transduce stimulation of neurotransmitter receptors into changes in intracellular activity and metabolism. Lithium does reduce the activity of the enzyme adenylate cyclase, which is normally activated when β-adrenoceptors are stimulated by noradrenaline. Indeed lithium induced renal and thyroid gland side-effects are linked to changes in the activity of adenylate cyclase.

In particular, the second messenger system that seems to be altered by lithium is the phosphatidylinositol (PI) pathway. Lithium blocks the regeneration of PI which ultimately leads to the inhibition of InsP3 (the major calcium-releasing messenger) formation and blocking of many receptor-mediated effects (Rang et al 1995). It has been suggested that this, for example, may lead to downregulation of an overactive dopamine system, leading to clinical improvement (Trimble 1996). There has been speculation that dopamine receptor hypersensitivity is closely associated with the onset of mania (Leonard 1997) and lithium does seem to reduce the hypersensitivity of both pre- and postsynaptic dopamine receptors (Leonard 1997). This could explain the mood-stabilising effects of lithium.

Lithium is also associated with β-adrenoceptor downregulation and with enhanced release of serotonin into the synapse, which may produce secondary postsynaptic receptor adaptation. This would be consistent with the observation that lithium has antidepressant effects and can be particularly effective in therapy-resistant depression when combined with an MAOI or an SSRI.

Attention has also been given to the effect that lithium has on the inhibitory neurotransmitter GABA. There does appear to be some evidence that lithium enhances the release of GABA by desensitising presynaptic GABA receptors, thereby modifying the autoregulation of GABA release (Leonard 1997).

Case study 8.1

Mary, is a 33-year-old woman who has two children and a long history of bipolar affective disorder. Following the birth of her first child, Mary has experienced frequent mood swings. Since commencing lithium five years ago her mood has become more stabilised, with her mood swings now being less severe. Over the past two years she has developed marked polydipsia and has been drinking over 5 l of fluid each day. As a result the dosage of lithium has had to be steadily increased to keep levels within the therapeutic range. Three weeks ago, while she was elated in her mood and receiving intensive support she developed a urinary tract infection. Unbeknown to her primary carers Mary stopped drinking for approximately three days and developed acute signs of lithium toxicity. She became mildly confused, had slurred speech, was unsteady on her feet and had a marked hand tremor. She was admitted to hospital and was found to have toxic levels of lithium. She was treated with intravenous fluids and peritoneal dialysis. As a result her lithium levels slowly began to fall. Two weeks later she was commenced on a different mood stabiliser, carbamazepine, and reports feeling well.

Unwanted effects

Lithium salts have a number of unwanted effects (Box 8.2). A common side-effect includes gastrointestinal disturbance (nausea, vomiting and diarrhoea). This can be severe enough to affect compliance but tends to wane over time. Weight gain can also be troublesome. In addition to increasing food intake, lithium also affects the intermediary stages of glucose metabolism, resulting in enhanced lipid synthesis.

Unwanted effects also include the development of a fine tremor. Due to inhibition of the action of thyroid stimulating hormone, hypothyroidism, with or without a goitre, can occur. Polyuria and polydipsia are also features, as lithium seems to block the renal action of antidiuretic hormone. The long-term administration of lithium has been associated with changes in renal function. While the significance of this association has not been fully established, it is still prudent to monitor renal function regularly and it is recommended that individuals should only be maintained on lithium after three to five years if benefit persists.

The main concern with lithium is that toxicity can easily occur, and to avoid this, plasma lithium levels must be regularly checked. The current recommendation is to maintain the plasma lithium level within 0.4 and 1.0 mmol Li^+/l for samples taken 12 hours after the preceding dose. Higher levels may be required to treat acute hypomanic episodes. On the initiation of treatment or following any change in dosage, particularly an increase, plasma levels should be monitored weekly for four to six weeks and thereafter every three to six weeks. Overdosage with plasma concentrations over 1.5 mmol Li^+/l may be fatal. It is vital that health professionals should be able to recognise the signs/symptoms of toxicity (Box 8.3) and that individuals taking lithium should be educated to also recognise the development of lithium toxicity. The concurrent use of diuretics is hazardous and should be avoided as lithium toxicity is made worse by sodium depletion.

Box 8.2   Unwanted effects of lithium salts

Nausea
Vomiting
Diarrhoea
Weight gain
Polyuria and polydipsia
Fine tremor
Hypothyroidism
Goitre
Exacerbation of psoriasis
Kidney changes

Box 8.3 Signs and symptoms of lithium toxicity

Blurred vision
Increasing gastrointestinal disturbance
Muscle weakness
CNS disturbances: drowsiness
                     sluggishness
                     ataxia
                     dysarthria
                     seizures

Other drugs as mood stabilisers

For completeness, comment should be made about other drugs that may have a place in the management of bipolar disorders. Carbamazepine is indicated when lithium is ineffective. It seems to be particularly useful for individuals who have a rapid cycle with four or more affective episodes per year. Traditional antipsychotic drugs have been used clinically to treat bipolar disorders and with the emergence of atypical antipsychotic drugs with better side-effect profiles, interest in their use for bipolar affective disorders has increased (Frye et al 1998, Tohen & Zarate 1998). Clinical experience to date suggests that clozapine has greater anti-mania properties compared to antidepressants, whereas risperidone is the converse with greater antidepressant than anti-mania properties (Frye et al 1998).

DRUGS USED IN PSYCHOSES AND RELATED DISORDERS

Various drugs are used clinically to manage individuals with episodes of psychoses (see Table 8.1). Initially termed *neuroleptics* (literally meaning 'gripping the neurone') because they caused extrapyramidal, movement disorders, with the development of atypical forms, the term *antipsychotic* was adopted (Bond & Lader 1996). Several classical antipsychotic drugs have been used extensively since chlorpromazine was introduced in 1953. Antipsychotics are classified into phenothiazines, butryophenones, thioxanthines and other related forms. Chlorpromazine, thioridazine and trifluoperazine are examples of the various groups classified as phenothiazines and they differ according to the degree of sedation provided and the extent of antimuscarinic and extrapyramidal side-effects they produce. Haloperidol, droperidol and benperidol are examples of butyrophenones; they tend to have fewer sedative side-effects and fewer antimuscarinic effects but more pronounced extrapyramidal side-effects. Flupenthixol and zuclopenthixol are examples of thioxanthines. Developments over the past three decades include the emergence of long-acting depot formulations (e.g. flupenthixol, zuclopenthixol and fluphenazine) and in recent years 'atypical' antipsychotics, for example clozapine and risperidone, which produce fewer extrapyramidal side-effects. Indeed clozapine has been found to be effective in some individuals unresponsive to conventional antipsychotic drugs. Olanzapine, quetiapine and sertindole have also recently been introduced onto the market. A comprehensive review of the new drug treatments for schizophrenia and the implications for nursing is provided by Gray et al (1997), who also address the issue of the different side effect profiles of both the typical and atypical antipsychotic drugs.

Due to the discovery that traditional neuroleptics, such as chlorpromazine and haloperidol, are dopamine receptor antagonists, the hypothesis of an abnormality in the dopaminergic system emerged, explaining the pathophysiological basis of schizophrenia. To some extent, even with the emergence of neuroleptics that also bind to $5HT_2$ receptors, for example clozapine, risperidone, quetiapine and olanzapine, there is reasonable pharmacological evidence to support the dopamine hypothesis (Bond & Lader 1996, Leonard 1997, Scatton & Zivkovic 1984, Trimble 1996).

Dopamine hypothesis

This hypothesis emerged with the introduction of phenothiazines in the 1960s and was proposed in 1965. There seems to be general agreement that schizophrenia is the result of overactivity of dopamine transmission within the CNS and that neuroleptics modify dopamine transmission. There is strong evidence that neuroleptics act at dopamine receptors in the limbic system (Scatton & Zivkovic 1984) and that their pharmacological effects are most likely due to blockade of selective dopamine receptors, namely D_2 and D_4.

Some inconsistencies are still present in the dopamine hypothesis. Dopamine transmission is rapidly altered at the synapse by neuroleptics but clinical improvement has a time delay. As with antidepressants this may be explained by some adaptive effect in the dopaminergic system as a result of the acute dopamine blockade (Trimble 1996). Evidence supporting the dopamine hypothesis is largely indirect, based on pharmacological studies. 'Direct' studies aimed at providing biochemical evidence have been inconsistent. The amount of the dopamine metabolite homovanillic acid (HVA) present in the CSF and plasma of schizophrenic patients has tended to be low or normal, rather than (as would be expected) high (Rang et al 1995, Trimble 1996). Nevertheless there appears to be some evidence that decreased levels of HVA may be compatible with increased dopamine receptor sensitivity with subsequent decreased dopamine turnover (Trimble 1996, Zemlan et al 1985).

Alteration of dopaminergic transmission also varies between different regions in the brain. A review of studies examining D_2 receptors show increased binding of neuroleptics with receptors in the caudate nucleus (Clardy et al 1994) where increases in dopamine have been reported. With interest developing in the significance of the relatively newly discovered D_4 receptors (Liegeois et al 1998, Seeman et al 1993), there has been a modification in the dopamine hypothesis away from increased dopamine turnover to increased postsynaptic receptor function, with D_4 receptors being particularly important (Trimble 1996). Of increasing interest is the relative importance of binding to D_2 and $5HT_2$ receptors as a way of understanding the pathophysiology of schizophrenia, with the emergence of the atypical neuroleptics with combined $5HT_2/D_2$ antagonism (Remington & Kapur 1999).

Mechanism of action

As outlined above, antipsychotic drugs owe their effects to blockade of dopamine D_2 and possibly D_4 receptors. The main groups, phenothiazines (e.g. chlorpromazine), thioxanthenes (e.g. clopenthixol) and butyrophenones (e.g. haloperidol), show preference for blocking D_2 receptors rather than D_1 (Rang et al 1995). The newer atypical neuroleptics differ in their selectivity. Clozapine is more selective for D_1 than D_2 receptors and has a high affinity for D_4 receptors. Risperidone has high affinity for D_2 and D_4 receptors. Olanzapine also has a high affinity for D_4 occupancy. All the drugs show greater $5HT_2$ than D_2 occupancy at all doses (Kapur et al 1999); although the difference is greatest for clozapine.

Case study 8.2

Alison is a 28-year-old woman with young children, who has a bipolar affective disorder. She mainly experiences severe hypomanic mood swings. Recently, in order to attempt to improve her compliance, Alison was commenced on a depot injection of Depixol. Following the second depot injection she began to develop oculogyric crises that would last for up to two hours each time. These episodes were extremely distressing, resulting in her having to sit down and being unable to see due to her eyes turning upward. She was commenced on procyclidine which she continues to take regularly. Four months later the oculogyric crises continue, although they are now much less frequent and they only occur when she stops taking her procyclidine. Investigations including a brain CT scan were all normal.

Unwanted effects

Antipsychotic drugs are also antagonistic at various other receptor types, for example α-adrenergic receptors, muscarinic (cholinergic) receptors,

---

Box 8.4 The common side-effects of antipsychotic drugs

Cardiovascular: postural hypotension (particularly phenothiazines and clozapine)

Extrapyramidal motor disturbance: parkinsonism-like symptoms

> tardive dyskinesia

Sedation

Weight gain

Antimuscarinic effects: dry mouth
constipation
blurred vision
difficulty with micturition

Endocrine disturbance: gynaecomastia
lactation
menstrual disturbances

Impotence

Haematological disturbance: leucopenia and agranulocytosis, particularly with
clozapine

Idiosyncratic and hypersensitive reactions: jaundice
skin reactions
neuroleptic malignant syndrome

$5HT_2$ receptors and histamine (H_1) receptors, which account for some of the unwanted and additional effects. The major unwanted effects are listed in Box 8.4. Motor disturbance (extrapyramidal) symptoms are the most troublesome and are related to the antagonistic action on dopamine. The two major forms are:

- parkinsonism-like symptoms
- tardive dyskinesia.

Parkinsonism-like symptoms Parkinsonism-like symptoms, including tremor and rigidity, are thought to be due to blocking dopamine activity within the nigrostriatal pathway of the basal ganglia. The symptoms are dose related, develop quite rapidly and are reversible on withdrawal of treatment. Symptoms may also be suppressed by the administration of antimuscarinic drugs, such as benzhexol, benztropine, orphenadrine and procyclidine. In the corpus striatal region of the basal ganglia, D_2 receptors inhibit the release of acetylcholine, therefore it is believed that parkinsonism-like motor abnormalities produced by neuroleptics may be due to excessive release of acetylcholine, hence the use of antimuscarinic drugs. It is worth noting that clozapine and risperidone have marked antimuscarinic effects and therefore movement disorders are not major side-effects with both drugs. Seeman & Tallerico (1998) further suggest that antipsychotic drugs that produce little or no parkinsonism, such as clozapine, do so because they bind more loosely than dopamine to D_2 receptors compared to antipsychotic drugs that do produce parkinsonism-like symptoms.

Tardive dyskinesia (TD) TD is a more serious form of movement disorder which is characterised by involuntary movements of the tongue, lips, cheeks and face, often combined with choreiform movements of the trunk and limbs. TD is associated with the chronic administration of neuroleptics, can occur when neuroleptics are stopped and is often very disabling and, so far, despite the investigation of various drugs, treatment still has limited success (Egan et al 1997). The incidence has been estimated at 20–40% of neuroleptic-treated patients (Cardosa & Jankovic 1997, Casey 1998, Rang et al 1995) but it depends on the neuroleptic used, as atypical neuroleptics such as clozapine and olanzapine have a low incidence of associated TD (Casey 1998, Kane 1999).

The reason why there is a lower incidence of TD with clozapine is not clear. Clozapine has a high affinity for D_1 and D_4 receptors thus producing relatively less blocking of the corpus striatal D_2 receptors. This coupled with its marked antimuscarinic activity may counteract any effect on the motor system. There is some evidence that TD may be associated with an increase in the number of D_2 postsynaptic receptors in the corpus striatum (Jenner & Marsden 1988). Although the reasons are not fully understood, neuroleptics that are less likely to cause TD also cause less receptor proliferation and dopamine supersensitivity (Rang et al 1995). Reduction in GABA levels within the basal ganglia may also be involved in the development of TD (Trimble 1996). There is increasing evidence that clozapine, because of its favourable motor effect profile, may be beneficial for individuals who suffer from or may develop TD (Casey 1998)

There appear to be a number of predisposing factors, including age (individuals over the age of 50 are more predisposed), gender (females are more predisposed) and early susceptibility to drug-induced parkinsonism-like symptoms. Individuals with schizophrenia who have more pronounced positive symptoms seem to be less likely to develop TD (Trimble 1996).

Other unwanted effects Due to the α-adrenergic blocking action of most typical neuroleptics, hypotension can be a problem. Of the atypical neuroleptics, clozapine also produces hypotension. Increased prolactin secretion due to dopamine D_2 receptor blocking can lead to breast enlargement and lactation in both women and men.

Idiosyncratic and hypersensitivity reactions Jaundice may occur with the older typical phenothiazines. The jaundice is the obstructive form and is usually mild but the exact mechanism for the hepatotoxicity is not clear. The jaundice clears when the drug is stopped or a neuroleptic of a different class is substituted. Leucopenia and agranulocytosis, while rare, are potentially life threatening. Chlorpromazine was associated with the development of agranulocytosis. In recent years clozapine has been found to have a much higher incidence (1–2%) of drug-induced leucopenia (Rang et al 1995). At present, all patients treated with clozapine (trade name Clozaril) need to be registered with the Clozaril Patient Monitoring Service and during the first 18 weeks of treatment leucocyte and differential blood counts need to be monitored weekly. Thereafter the recommendation is that blood counts are monitored fortnightly. The monitoring of the white blood cell count is not reduced in frequency until patients have been receiving treatment for a year or more and have had stable blood counts.

Neuroleptic malignant syndrome is rare but it has been linked to haloperidol, chlorpromazine and flupenthixol decanoate. Cases attributed to clozapine and risperidone have also been reported (Hasan & Buckley 1998). This is a serious extrapyramidal complication, presenting as hyperthermia, muscular rigidity and autonomic disturbance. Tachycardia, pallor, sweating, labile blood pressure and urinary incontinence may feature and death may occur from respiratory, cardiac, hepatic or renal failure. In view of the high mortality associated with neuroleptic malignant syndrome (10–20% of cases) and the fact that it can occur very rapidly, mental health nurses and other health care professionals need to be vigilant in observing for any early signs. Discontinuation of the neuroleptic is essential and the syndrome may last five to 10 days following discontinuation. Indeed this may be longer if a depot preparation is used. Overall, mental health nurses need to be well versed and efficient in the use of specific rating scales for the detection of side-effects such as the Barnes rating scale for drug-induced akathisia (Barnes 1989).

Treatment resistance

Treatment resistance has always been a problem for some individuals and as many as 10–45% of individuals receiving antipsychotic drugs may suffer from it (Meltzer 1997). Resistance of negative symptoms and cognitive function to antipsychotic drugs seems to be present following the first acute episode and does not evolve over time to the same extent as resistance of positive symptoms (Meltzer et al 1998). Clozapine seems to have an important place in the management of individuals with treatment resistance (Palmer et al 1999). The lifetime suicide rate in both treatment-resistant and responsive schizophrenic individuals is 9–13% (Meltzer 1997) and for individuals who have persistent suicidal thoughts, when treated with clozapine, the potential decrease in suicide is estimated to be as high as 85% (Meltzer 1998). Interestingly a recent survey in Finland identified 57% of suicide victims with active-phase schizophrenia were prescribed inadequate neuroleptic treatment or were non-compliant (Helia et al 1999).

Case study 8.3

Tony is a 30-year-old man who has suffered from schizophrenia for 12 years. He is extremely intelligent and, despite treatment with large doses of traditional neuroleptics, including depot preparations, he continued to experience auditory hallucinations both day and night. A crisis was reached two years ago when he decided that he could no longer cope with the constant haranguing and critical voices and decided to kill himself. He lay in a bath of cold water and cut his throat. He was found about one hour later by his parents and was rushed to casualty. He subsequently spent several weeks in an intensive care unit. Over the following months he made a full recovery from his attempted suicide but continued to hallucinate actively. At this stage he was commenced on clozapine tablets and over the following five to six weeks in hospital the hallucinatory experiences began to diminish for the first time in 12 years. Unfortunately, while he was experiencing considerable improvement in his 'symptoms', as he always described them, he also began to develop side-effects from the clozapine, including a marked stammer that made it impossible for him to communicate. However, despite this side-effect, he expressed a preference to remain on the medication.

As the new atypical drugs were introduced, Tony was commenced on olanzapine and in addition Seroquel tablets. On his current combination at a very high dosage (olanzapine 90 mg per day and Seroquel 800 mg daily), he has experienced an almost complete remission of his auditory hallucinations. He and his parents reported that he had not been as well as this for at least 12 years and he has now moved out of the family home and lives independently. He continues on high doses of atypical medication. In such cases clinical accountability lies with the consultant psychiatrist and not the drug manufacturer.

DRUGS USED FOR ANXIETY

Anxiety is a common human experience. Furthermore, anxiety is a feature of several mental health problems but as a condition in itself anxiety may take the form of generalised anxiety disorder, panic attacks, phobias, obsessive–compulsive disorder or post-traumatic stress disorder. When anxiety becomes disabling then anxiolytics can be of help. Anxiolytics have traditionally included barbiturates, but while there may still be a place for barbiturates in the management of epilepsy, they will not be discussed within the context of this chapter. Benzodiazepines (BZDs) and serotonin agonists are the main focus of this section. BZDs include chlordiazepoxide, diazepam, alprazolam, lorazepam and oxazepam which are shorter acting. As well as being anxiolytics, BZDs also have hypnotic, muscle relaxant and anticonvulsant properties.

Anxiolytics: mode of action

Benzodiazepines

It is only during the past two decades that the mode of action of BZDs has become clear. BZDs modulate inhibitory nerve transmission within the brain via GABA receptors. They do not act directly on GABA receptors but bind to receptor sites linked to the inhibitory $GABA_A$-chloride complex (Bond & Lader 1996). Diazepam binding in the brain shows a distinctive pattern, with the greatest binding occurring in the cerebral cortex and less in the limbic system and brainstem (Rang et al 1995). This is consistent with the location of $GABA_A$ receptors. The interaction between the BZD receptor and $GABA_A$ subunits is very complex and is still not completely understood. Indeed multiple potential configurations of the BZD-GABA receptor exist. In essence BZDs enhance the normal GABA-mediated inhibition by binding to BZD receptors.

It is worth noting that the presence of BZD receptors in the brain would suggest that naturally occurring 'BZD' chemicals exist, in the same way as endorphins bind to opiate receptors. However, no single specific compound has been identified, although a number of possible compounds have been isolated that show agonist or inverse agonist activity (Leonard 1997).

Serotonin agonists

Interest has also focused on other neurotransmitters that are modified via the GABA pathway, notably serotonin. Buspirone has high affinity for $5HT_{1A}$ receptors, which are located abundantly in the septohippocampal region of the brain (Rang et al 1995). How 5HT agonists exert the anxiolytic effects remains unclear. In contrast to BZDs, buspirone lacks hypnotic, muscle relaxant and anticonvulsant properties, and at high concentrations it acts as an antidepressant. As an anxiolytic, buspirone is both equipotent and equieffective with diazepam, but the onset of activity is slower than with conventional BZDs. Increasingly buspirone is being used in the management of disorders other than general anxiety disorder including obsessive–compulsive disorder, post-traumatic stress disorder and panic disorders (Apter & Allen 1999).

Anxiolytics: unwanted effects

BZDs have very different unwanted effects compared to 5HT agonists: confusion, drowsiness, amnesia and impaired motor performance are the main side-effects of BZDs; however, the main effects with 5HT agonists are nausea, dizziness, headache and restlessness.

Dependence and withdrawal

Early claims that BZDs do not produce dependence have now been refuted. BZDs must be withdrawn gradually as abrupt withdrawal may produce confusion and convulsions. The BZD withdrawal syndrome is characterised by insomnia, anxiety, loss of appetite and weight loss, tremor, perspiration, tinnitus and perceptual disturbance and may occur anywhere from within a few hours of stopping a short-acting BZD up to three weeks after cessation.

PSYCHOPHARMACOLOGY AND ELDERLY PEOPLE

Particular care must be taken when using psychotropic drugs in elderly people. There is general agreement that older people will experience more adverse effects from psychotropic drugs. Individuals over the age of 70 years may experience nearly twice as many drug reactions as those under the age of 50 (Leonard 1997). BZDs, for example, are more likely to produce dizziness, which can lead to falls and serious injury. The increased sensitivity of some older people to the sedating effects of many psychotropic drugs, particularly anxiolytics, is well known. It is therefore prudent to consider the use of drugs with a short half-life. The hypotensive effects of antidepressants and phenothiazine neuroleptics may be increased in older people, particularly if they have a tendency to be dehydrated. This may lead to postural hypotension and falls, thus compromising their safety.

In general, with regard to pharmacodynamics, drug metabolism is much slower and elimination of drugs is reduced in elderly people. This necessitates the initial use of lower doses with a slower increase of the dose to achieve optimal benefit.

CONCLUSION

Used alongside other appropriate interventions, drug treatment can dramatically improve the quality of life of an individual with mental health problems and enable him/her to function purposefully within society and within personal relationships. Psychopharmacology is a growing area. As fast as the understanding of how drugs act on the brain increases, the more the limits of understanding become apparent. New drugs are entering the clinical arena at a rapid pace and it is likely that future developments will further expand the range of drugs on offer for clinicians to choose from. This chapter is not meant to be an all-inclusive, up-to-date list of the drugs available; its purpose is to identify the various groups of drugs that may be used in the treatment of individuals with specific mental health problems and to outline the mechanisms by which neuronal transmission can be modified in the brain to produce mental health benefit.

It is up to individual mental health nurses and other health professionals and key workers to keep themselves abreast of new drugs as they emerge into the clinical arena. Furthermore, as well as increasing their knowledge of all types of medication, including side-effects, mental health nurses need to develop skills in recognising and managing noncompliance, assessing clinical symptoms and the use of various drug educational strategies (Gray et al 1997).

REFERENCES

Apter J T, Allen L A 1999 Buspirone: future directions. Journal of Clinical Psychopharmacology 19: 86–93

Barnes T R E 1989 A rating scale for drug induced akathisia. British Journal of Psychiatry 154: 672–676

Benedetti M S, Dostert P 1992 Monoamine oxidase: from physiology and pathophysiology to the design and clinical application of reversible inhibitors. Advances in Drug Research 23: 66–125

Bond A J, Lader M H 1996 Understanding drug treatment in mental health care. Wiley, Chichester

Cardosa F, Jankovic J 1997 Dystonia and dyskinesia. Psychiatric Clinics of North America 20: 821–838

Casey D E 1998 Effects of clozapine therapy in schizophrenic individuals at risk for tardive dyskinesia. Journal of Clinical Psychiatry 59(suppl 3): 31–37

Clardy J A, Hyde T M, Kleinman J E 1994 Post-mortem neurochemical and neuropathological studies in schizophrenia. In: Andreasen N (ed) Schizophrenia from mind to molecule. American Psychiatric Association Press, Washington

Egan M F, Apud J, Wyatt R J 1997 Treatment of tardive dyskinesia. Schizophrenia Bulletin 23: 583–609

Frye M A, Ketter T A, Altshuler L L et al 1998 Clozapine in bipolar disorder: treatment implications for other atypical antipsychotics. Journal of Affective Disorders 48: 91–104

Gray R, Gournay K, Taylor D 1997 New drug treatments for schizophrenia: implications for mental health nursing. Mental Health Practice 1(1): 20–23

Hasan S, Buckley P 1998 Novel antipsychotics and the neuroleptic syndrome: a review and critique. American Journal of Psychiatry 155: 1113–1116

Helia H, Isometsa E T, Henriksson M M, Heikkinen M E, Marttunen M J, Lonnqvist J K 1999 Suicide victims with schizophrenia in different phases of adequacy of antipsychotic medication. Journal of Clinical Psychiatry 60: 200–208

Jenner P, Marsden C D 1988 Adaptive changes in brain dopamine function as a result of neuroleptic treatment. Advances in Neurology 49: 417–431

Kane J M 1999 Tardive dyskinesia in affective disorders. Journal of Psychiatry 60(suppl 5): 43–47

Kapur S, Zipursky R B, Remington G 1999 Clinical and theoretical implications of 5HT2 and D2 receptor occupancy of clozapine, risperidone and olanzapine in schizophrenia. American Journal of Psychiatry 156: 286–293

Leonard B E 1997 Fundamentals of psychopharmacology, 2nd edn. Wiley, Chichester

Liegeois J, Eyrolles L, Bruhwyler J, Delarge J 1998 Dopamine D4 receptors: a new opportunity for research on schizophrenia. Current Medicinal Chemistry 5: 77–100

Meltzer H Y 1997 Treatment-resistant schizophrenia – the role of clozapine. Current Medical Research and Opinion 14: 1–20

Meltzer H Y 1998 Suicide in schizophrenia: risk factors and clozapine treatment. Journal of Clinical Psychiatry 59(suppl 3): 15–20

Meltzer H Y, Lee M, Cola P 1998 The evolution of treatment resistance: biologic implications. Journal of Clinical Psychopharmacology 18(2 suppl 1): 5S–11S

Montigny C De, Blier P 1985 Electrophysiological aspects of serotonin neuropharmacology. In: Green A R (ed) Neuropharmacology of serotonin. Oxford University Press, Oxford, p 181

Palmer D D, Henter I D, Wyatt R J 1999 Do antipsychotic medications decrease the risk of suicide in patients with schizophrenia? Journal of Clinical Psychiatry 60(suppl 2): 100–103

Rang H P, Dale M M, Ritter J M 1995 Pharmacology, 3rd edn. Churchill Livingstone, Edinburgh

Remington G, Kapur S 1999 D2 and 5HT2 receptor effects of antipsychotics: bridging basic and clinical findings using PET. Journal of Clinical Psychiatry 60(suppl 10): 15–19

Scatton B, Zivkovic B 1984 Neuroleptics and the limbic system. In: Trimble M R, Zarifian E (eds) Psychopharmacology of the limbic system. Oxford University Press, Oxford, p 124

Seeman P, Tallerico T 1998 Antipsychotic drugs which elicit little or no parkinsonism bind more loosely than dopamine to D2 receptors, yet occupy high levels of these receptors. Molecular Psychiatry 3: 123–134

Seeman P, Guan H C, Vantol H M M 1993 Dopamine D4 receptors elevated in schizophrenia. Nature 365: 441–445

Sulser F 1984 Regulation and function of noradrenaline receptor in systems in brain. Neurophamacology 23: 255–261

Tohen M, Zarate C A Jr 1998 Antipsychotic agents and bipolar disorders. Journal of Clinical Psychiatry 59(suppl 1): 38–48

Trimble M R 1996 Biological psychiatry, 2nd edn. Wiley, Chichester

Zemlan F P, Hitzemann R J, Hirschowitz J, Garver D L 1985 Down regulation of central dopamine receptors in schizophrenia. American Journal of Psychiatry 142: 1334–1337

9

Sleep and sensory functioning

Key Points

- The quality rather than the amount of sleep is important for good health and social/behavioural functioning
- The function of sleep remains a subject of much debate
- Sleep seems to be a restorative process particularly orientated towards restitution of the brain
- Only approximately 33% of total sleep loss is recovered and this is largely slow wave sleep
- Sleep disturbance can be an early indicator of the development of mental health problems
- Shortened REM latency has a high sensitivity and specificity in depression
- Newer non-benzodiazepine hypnotics are reported to produce less daytime sedation and cognitive impairment
- Hypnotics should not be the first line of treatment for sleep disorders
- Narcolepsy is a disorder of REM sleep control and requires long-term management

There is general agreement that sleep, of a good quality, is important for good health and effective social/behavioural functioning. Indeed, it is well recognised that alterations in sleep pattern are one of the earliest indicators of mental distress. It is therefore of value for mental health nurses and health professionals to understand the nature and importance of sleep. Simplistically, it is not the quantity of sleep that is crucial, but the quality. Within this chapter, sleep as a physiological phenomenon and the function of sleep are discussed. Alterations in the pattern of sleep associated with specific mental health problems are also considered. Finally the use of hypnotic drugs to promote sleep is discussed.

SLEEP ARCHITECTURE

In humans, using polysomnographs, two main types of sleep have been identified:

- rapid eye movement (REM) sleep
- non-rapid eye movement sleep (non-REM sleep or slow wave sleep).

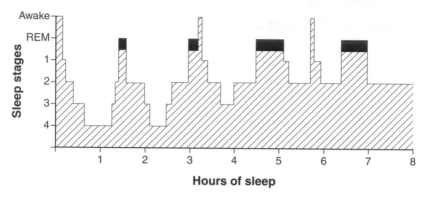

Figure 9.1 Typical polysomnogram for a young adult. From Horne, by permission of Oxford University Press. 1988

Normal sleep involves several cycles of REM and non-REM sleep. Figure 9.1 shows a normal pattern of sleep for a young adult. As illustrated, the typical sleep pattern shows four key features of sleep (Horne 1988):

- a rapid descent to stage 4 following the onset of sleep
- a regular 90–minute cycle of REM sleep and other stages
- the prevalence of stages 3 and 4 (slow wave sleep) in the first cycle then progressively less during subsequent cycles
- a greater predominance of REM sleep and stage 2 sleep in the second half of sleep.

Typically, individuals first go into non-REM sleep, descending from stage 1 through to stage 4 sleep. During this phase, electroencephalograph (EEG) waves become slower and their amplitude greater. The depth of sleep then returns to stage 2, following which, the first episode of REM sleep occurs. Typically, sleep consists of four to six cycles of non-REM sleep alternating with REM sleep. Each repeating cycle is approximately 90 minutes in length, with each cycle containing 20- to 30-minute bouts of REM sleep. As illustrated, stages 3 and 4 are more pronounced during the early part of the sleep period and the duration of REM sleep increases as sleep progresses.

Non-REM sleep

Non-REM sleep is divided into light sleep (stages 1 and 2) and delta or slow wave sleep (stages 3 and 4). Stage 1 sleep is characterised by the appearance of theta rhythm on the EEG (Fig. 9.2) and forms the transition between wakefulness and sleep. It occupies approximately 5% of the total sleep time (Horne 1988). Muscle tone is relatively weak and while a certain amount of mental activity persists, concentration and

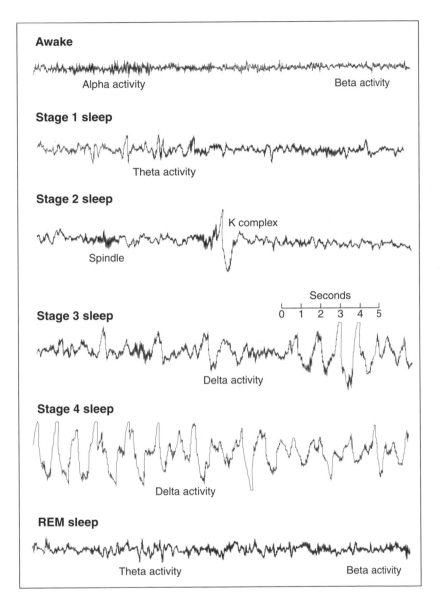

Figure 9.2 Typical EEG waveforms during the various sleep stages. From Horne, by permission of Oxford University Press. 1988

imagination fluctuate. Hypnagogic hallucinations may occur as the sleep deepens.

Stage 2 sleep accounts for over 50% of the total sleep time and is marked by characteristic sleep spindles and K complexes on the EEG (Horne 1988). Sleep spindles are short bursts of waves of 12–14 Hz that occur between two and five times per minute during stages 1–4. The significance of these is not fully understood but it is suggested that sleep spindles represent the activity of a mechanism that decreases the sensitivity of the brain to sensory input and thus maintains sleep (Bowersox et al 1985). K complexes are sudden, sharp complexes which are only found during stage 2 sleep. They seem to occur spontaneously at a rate of approximately one per minute and can be triggered by noise, and they may also represent neuronal activity directed at keeping the person asleep (Halasz et al 1985).

Occasionally during stage 2 sleep, delta waves may be present. Muscle tone is weak and there are no eye movements. Although a person may be 'sleeping soundly' during this stage of sleep, if awakened they may report that they were not asleep but awake.

Stages 3 and 4 (slow wave sleep) account for approximately 20% of total sleep time. Delta waves predominate in the EEG. The distinction between stage 3 and 4 sleep is not so clear. Stage 3 contains approximately 20–50% delta activity while stage 4 sleep delta activity is greater than 50% (Carlson 1994, Horne 1988). This stage is associated with growth hormone secretion and tissue repair. Dreaming may occur but it is usually of a brief duration and of a rational nature. Nocturnal terrors and sleep-walking are associated with this stage.

REM sleep

REM sleep occupies approximately 20% of the normal sleep time for a young adult. In young children it is higher at 30% and in older people much reduced at less than 20%. The EEG pattern resembles that of wakefulness but there is muscular relaxation. This type of sleep is characterised by short bursts of rapid eye movement with sporadic muscular twitches of the face and extremities. While there is skeletal muscle relaxation there is activation of the autonomic system with hypertension, tachycardia alternating with bradycardia and, in males, penile erection. Cortisol secretion seems to peak at the end of the sleep cycle when REM sleep is most pronounced. Typically in the EEG, 4 Hz 'sawtooth' waves occur near the onset of REM sleep.

FUNCTION OF SLEEP

This has been the subject of much debate and conjecture. There is reasonable evidence, mainly from animal studies and to a lesser extent from human studies, that sleep is a restorative process (Oswald 1987), particularly orientated towards restitution of the brain (Horne 1988). Slow wave (stage 4) sleep, is associated with peak levels of growth hormone. Growth hormone stimulates protein synthesis, the uptake of amino acids and tissue restoration. Anabolic processes seem to be a feature of slow wave sleep, but the significance of this is unclear as the plasma level of amino acids during sleep is normally low.

Total sleep deprivation studies have not provided convincing evidence that sleep is needed to keep the body functioning normally (Carlson 1994). Sleep deprivation does not seem to produce a physiological stress response or interfere with the ability to perform physical exercise, but it does impair cognitive functioning. Perceptual distortions and hallucinations are often reported following 48 hours of total sleep deprivation. Further effects include behavioural irritability, suspiciousness and slurring of speech. Not all of the sleep that is deprived is reclaimed. Only approximately 33% of the total sleep loss is recovered and this is largely slow wave sleep. Approximately 50% of REM sleep is made up, with little of stage 1 and 2.

The precise function of REM sleep is unknown but it is associated with dreaming, where the dreams are long, emotional and animated. The evidence provided to explain the function of REM sleep is inconclusive. Various hypotheses have been proposed, including permitting the animal to become more sensitive to the environment and therefore avoid being surprised by predators, enhancing learning, integrating learned and instinctive behaviours and facilitating brain development (Carlson 1994).

Current opinion favours the facilitation of learning and memory, particularly where the newly learned information has emotional consequences. REM sleep and its associated dreaming may help the person to deal with specific learning experiences that involve an emotional component. REM sleep deprivation does seem to impair learning, especially of complicated tasks, but the effect is quite minor (Smith 1985). Furthermore, it has been demonstrated in college students that REM sleep increased at the time of examinations (Smith & Lapp 1991).

Where individuals experience REM sleep deprivation, there is a rebound effect. When permitted to sleep normally, individuals spend a greater than normal percentage of time in REM sleep, suggesting that REM sleep is both regulated and has an important function. Contrary to assumptions made during early sleep studies in the 1960s, REM sleep deprivation is not associated with the development of hallucinations and psychiatric symptoms.

PHYSIOLOGICAL BASIS OF SLEEP

It is now generally accepted that sleep and the level of arousal is modulated within the diffuse group of neurones that comprise the reticular formation. This region consists of parts of the medulla, pons and midbrain. Animal studies have demonstrated that lesions of the reticular formation result in somnolence and coma. Arousal from sleep by sensory stimuli is simplistically attributed to collateral pathways that link the main sensory pathways to the reticular formation.

A number of neurotransmitters appear to be involved in modulating sleep and wakefulness. Noradrenergic projections from the rostral part of the locus coeruleus (upper pons and midbrain region) seem to be involved in the maintenance of cortical arousal and the ascending cholinergic pathways (Carlson 1994, Leonard 1992). Acetylcholine also has an important role in modulating wakefulness and arousal. Many of the projections from the reticular formation to the thalamus and the basal forebrain are cholinergic (Carlson 1994). Furthermore, acetylcholine antagonists decrease EEG signs of cortical arousal (Vanderwolf 1992). Inhibition of the cholinergic pathways by GABA may be important in the regulation of REM sleep. It has been postulated that activation of $GABA_A$ receptors may play a crucial role in the initiation and maintenance of non-REM sleep and in the generation of sleep spindles (Lancel 1999).

Serotonin (5HT) also has a major role in the modulation of the sleep–wake pattern. Serotonin is largely located in the raphe nuclei, which are located in the medullary and pontine regions of the reticular formation. Stimulation of the raphe nuclei cause increased locomotion and cortical activity. Serotonergic neurones are most active during waking, with their firing rate declining during slow wave sleep. The activity of serotonergic neurones is almost non-existent during REM sleep, except for a brief pulse of activity immediately after the cessation of REM sleep (Carlson 1994).

Neural control of stage 4 (slow wave) sleep

Animal studies using cats and rats have demonstrated that an area of the brain just above the hypothalamus called the basal forebrain region seems to be important in regulating stage 4 sleep. Stimulation via electrical means or warming of the basal forebrain causes drowsiness and EEG changes consistent with sleepiness (Carlson 1994). McGinty & Szymusiak (1990) provided evidence that neurones in the temperature-regulating area of the hypothalamus (preoptic area) become active when the region is warmed artificially as well as when animals fall asleep. Indeed this may explain why we feel sleepy when it is hot. The suggestion is made that one function of slow wave sleep may be to reduce brain metabolism and therefore to allow the brain to cool (McGinty & Szymusiak 1990).

Neural control of REM sleep

As identified earlier, REM sleep is characterised by rapid eye movements, desynchronised EEG activity and muscular paralysis. In animals, activation of REM sleep seems to be located primarily within the pons and is dependent on the release of acetylcholine. The release of acetylcholine and activation of REM sleep is normally inhibited by the noradrenergic neurones of the locus coeruleus and the serotonergic neurones of the raphe nuclei. Acetylcholine agonists induce REM sleep. It has been proposed that the reduction in serotoninergic and noradrenergic neuronal activity is the trigger for REM sleep (Carlson 1994). However, the nature and location of a pacemaker that controls the cycle of REM and slow wave sleep is still not known. Indeed the question as to whether the sleep cycle is related to changes in the temperature of the brain has not been fully answered.

SLEEP AND CIRCADIAN RHYTHMS

Biological phenomena such as temperature, hormonal secretion and the immune system fluctuate over time in response to internal and external factors. Within organisms, biological activities that follow rhythms that repeat every 24 hours are called circadian rhythms (*circa* means 'about' and *dies* means 'day'). Circadian rhythms may be controlled by internal mechanisms (internal clock) and set or synchronised by rhythms external to the organism. A rhythm that is external to the organism is called a *zeitgeber* (German for 'time giver'). The sleep–wake cycle is an example of a circadian rhythm. Regular daily variation in light keeps the internal clock adjusted to 24 hours. Light serves as a *zeitgeber*; it sets the endogenous rhythm. As to the location of the 'internal clock'; in rats it is located in the suprachiasmatic nucleus (SCN) of the hypothalamus. Direct connections between the retina and the SCN have been demonstrated, which is consistent with the phenomenon that light sets the sleep–wake cycle. Glutamic acid and neuropeptide Y appear to be the neurotransmitters involved in the regulation of neuronal activity in the SCN by light. It seems reasonable that in humans the SCN may function as the internal clock, but how this regulates the sleep–wake cycle is not fully understood.

INSOMNIA

There is no single definition of insomnia. The significance of insomnia as a health problem may not be fully appreciated. It has been estimated that in any one year the incidence of insomnia is approximately 30% of the population, and only one in 256 patients with insomnia presents to their general practitioner (Shapiro & Dement 1993).

Sleep disorders may involve disorders of initiating and maintaining sleep (DIMS) and disorders of excessive somnolence (DOES). Insomnia is a subjective experience involving a perception of too much wakefulness and poor quality of sleep related to:

- difficulty in initiating sleep (DIS)
- difficulty in maintaining sleep (DMS)
- difficulty in initiating and maintaining sleep (DIMS)

With regard to the use of hypnotics, insomnia may be classified as:

- Transient insomnia: this may occur in normal sleepers and may be due to extraneous factors such as shift pattern changes, jet lag or acute stressful events.
- Short-term insomnia: this is usually associated with situational stress such as that resulting from a serious medical illness, unemployment, bereavement or family conflict; it may last for a few weeks and may recur.
- Long-term (chronic) insomnia: the cause of this is often multifactorial. This form of insomnia in up to 50% of individuals is related to an underlying mental health disorder, such as depression (Leonard 1992). The remaining factors include chronic alcohol and drug abuse.

SLEEP AND AFFECTIVE DISORDER

Some disorder of sleep is a common and well-established symptom of depression. A summary of the major disorders of sleep associated with depression is presented in Table 9.1. Clinically there is held a view that waking early in the morning is linked to endogenous depression. Based

---

Case study 9.1

Jack is 32 years of age, lives with his parents and is a keen electric guitarist. He has suffered from a schizophrenic illness which has led to a pattern of admission to hospital every year for the past eight years. He has very little insight into his condition and as soon as he is discharged from hospital he discontinues all his medication. While on neuroleptic medication he appears very well, is quite spontaneous, relates very well to his parents and helps them in the garden centre where they work. At this time he has a normal sleep–wake cycle and drinks very little alcohol.

After approximately two to three months following discharge from hospital and Jack not taking his medication, his sleep–wake pattern begins to alter. He begins to be awake for longer periods during the night and to sleep at times during the day. Gradually he becomes more active during the night and plays his music through the night, much to the distress of his parents. His alcohol intake during this period increases, and frequent arguments between Jack and his mother, who find his behaviour quite unacceptable, begin to occur. As his mental state deteriorates he becomes more paranoid, accusing neighbours of staring at him and also of broadcasting his thoughts. He starts to become convinced of some mystical force surrounding the house and believes that the neighbours are listening to all of his conversations. As Jack continues to deteriorate his sleep–wake cycle completely reverses, he actively hallucinates and becomes socially isolated from his parents. It is at this time that he requires formal admission to hospital and the cycle then repeats.

Case study 9.2

Irene is a 53-year-old woman who developed a psychotic illness for the first time about four years ago. She hears voices when she is not treated with neuroleptics. Investigations at the time of her original admission to hospital showed that she had mild weakness in one hand and a CT brain scan and NMR scan showed that she had small plaques in the hindbrain and brainstem. A lumbar puncture at that time showed CSF immunoglobulin suggestive of multiple sclerosis.

Following treatment of her psychotic illness she has returned home where she lives by herself and has an active social life. She no longer has any weakness in her hands but complains bitterly that she is totally unable to sleep and has lost all sense of taste and smell. Large dosages of neuroleptics or hypnotics have no effect on her and attempts to record a sleep EEG have so far failed as she has remained alert even when sedated with amylobarbitone. She reports that through the night she watches night-time television and listens to music but that she gets extremely bored in the early hours of the morning. She is bright and alert during the day and there appear to be no signs of any mood disturbance. It seems highly likely that this sleep disturbance is due to organic degenerative processes.

Table 9.1 Major disorders of sleep associated with depression

Aspect of sleep	Sleep problem
Reported symptoms	Difficulty getting off to sleep Poor sleep Early morning waking Increased waking
Duration	Decreased total time
Non-REM sleep	Increased stage 1 Decreased stages 3 and 4
REM sleep	Decreased REM latency Increased REM time in early hours Decreased REM in late hours

Modified from Trimble (1996). Copyright John Wiley & Sons Limited
Reproduced with permission.

on polysomnographically defined sleep changes, one consistent observation has been decreased REM latency, i.e. the time from the onset of sleep to the first REM period (Thase 1998). Trimble (1996) reported that this falls by approximately 30% and is associated with an increase in length of the first REM period, decreases in stage 3 and 4 sleep and increased waking periods during the night.

While shortened REM latency is not specific for depression it does have a very high sensitivity and specificity (Thase 1998, Trimble 1996). Benca et al (1992) conducted a meta-analysis of sleep disorders and confirmed that while a reduction in total sleep time was associated with a number of mental illness conditions, this was largely due to decreases in non-REM sleep. This is in contrast to depression where the percentage of REM sleep was increased.

The meaning of these changes is unclear. As they are commonly linked to a form of depression termed endogenous depression, the pattern of early waking and increased REM sleep may reflect the underlying biochemical disturbance. A deficit of serotonergic neurotransmission, a relative increase in pontine cholinergic activity and possibly an excess of noradrenergic activity have been implicated in the pathogenesis of sleep disturbances associated with severe depression (Thase 1998).

Acute and serious elevation of mood associated with schizophrenia and bipolar disorders may also result in alteration of the sleep–wake cycle. An inability to rest, agitation, overactivity and fear associated with paranoid thoughts may result in prolonged periods of wakefulness and an inability to fall asleep. Ultimately sleep time may be reduced significantly and there may be reversal of the sleep–wake pattern

SLEEP AND DELIRIUM

Delirium is a reversible confusional state with rapid onset. Symptoms of delirium appear over hours and days and include cognitive impairment, alterations in level of consciousness, perceptual disturbance and disorientation in time, place and person. Delirium is more common in older people due to increased susceptibility to brain hypoxia, underlying or existing organic brain damage and increased susceptibility to adverse drug reactions. The causes of delirium include infectious agents, toxins/drugs, metabolic abnormalities, trauma, central nervous system (CNS) pathology, cerebral ischaemia and hypoxaemia. Evening agitation and overactivity may be contrasted with daytime sleeping. Reversal of the sleep–wake cycle is a common feature. It is important to treat the underlying cause of the delirium. Hypnotics may have a place but alternative strategies to focus any agitation and to help restore the normal sleep–wake cycle should be attempted.

SLEEP AND ELDERLY PEOPLE

Sleep patterns and times show a number of changes over the lifespan. There is a general trend for a reduction in REM sleep and the total sleep time with advancing age. Indeed, older people tend to sleep less but spend longer in bed, have comparatively less stage 4 and REM sleep and have more shifts between sleep stages.

It seems that insomnia affects 25–35% of people over the age of 65 years (Brabbins et al 1993) and the problem tends to be one of sleep maintenance rather than difficulty in the initiation of sleep. Interestingly, the intensity of noise required to arouse a person from sleep decreases with age. This reduction is evident in all stages of sleep but is most significant in stage 4 slow wave sleep. Noise can lead to increased periods of wakening and poor sleep, and therefore attention needs to be given to the reduction of noise by health care workers. Increased noise, increased anxiety, pain and the unfamiliar surroundings of a new environment are factors that can result in poor-quality sleep and sleep deprivation for older people. Coupled with disorientation arising from dementia or toxic factors, sleeplessness may be increased, leading to increased activity in the evening and night with reversal of the sleep–wake cycle.

SLEEP AND THE USE OF HYPNOTICS

Many of the anxiolytic drugs identified in Chapter 8 can also be used as hypnotics. Benzodiazepines, such as nitrazepam, flurazepam, flunitrazepam and temazepam have traditionally been used as hypnotics. Newer non-benzodiazepine compounds, such as zopiclone and zolpidem, have emerged with added benefits of having short action and being devoid of any residual daytime sedation in low doses. Other compounds are also still used, such as chloral derivatives, chlormethiazole, antihistamines and sedative antidepressants. Chloral hydrate and triclofos were used for children but the use of hypnotics in children is not usually justified and there is now no real convincing evidence that chloral derivatives have a use as hypnotics. Chlormethiazole may be useful for elderly people as it does not produce hangover effects, but dependency can occur with long-term use, so routine administration is undesirable.

The choice of a hypnotic requires consideration of the rapidity of onset of action, the duration of action (see Table 9.2), the degree of daytime residual sedation (hangover effects) and the extent of rebound following discontinuation.

Hypnotics should be used selectively and should not be prescribed indiscriminately. They should be reserved for short-term use only and their use should be avoided as far as possible in elderly people, where the risk of causing dizziness and falls is too great. If they are indicated

Table 9.2 Duration and half-life of selected hypnotics

Hypnotic	Duration and half-life of selected hypnotics Half-life ($t_{1/2}$) (hours)	Duration of action
Flurazepam	48–120	Long
Nitrazepam	25–35	Long
Temazepam	8–20	Intermediate
Zolpidem	1.5–2.5	Short
Zopiclone	5–6	Short

Modified from Bond & Lader (1996). Copyright John Wiley & Sons Limited. Reproduced with permission.

for transient insomnia, a hypnotic that is rapidly eliminated should be selected and it should be restricted to one or two doses. Even in the treatment of short-term insomnia it is recommended that treatment should be restricted to between one and three weeks (preferably only one week), with an intermittent pattern of use where on selected days the hypnotic is omitted.

HYPNOTICS AND SLEEP ARCHITECTURE

All hypnotics, except zolpidem, alter the sleep architecture. Generally they alter both REM phase and non-REM sleep. Benzodiazepine hypnotics tend to (Dujardin et al 1998, Leonard 1992):

- reduce the quantity and quality of REM sleep
- suppress stage 3 and 4 sleep
- decrease stage 1 and prolong stage 2 sleep.

Compared to flunitrazepam, zolpidem does not alter sleep architecture (Dujardin et al 1998).

HYPNOTICS: UNWANTED SIDE-EFFECTS

The side-effect profile does vary between benzodiazepine and non-benzodiazepine hypnotics (see Box 9.1). Adverse effects such as daytime sedation, amnesia and depression are strongly dose related. The main concerns over the use of hypnotics relate to:

- residual effects
- rebound and withdrawal.

Box 9.1 Major unwanted effects from hypnotics

Benzodiazepine hypnotics: drowsiness and lightheadedness (next day)
confusion and ataxia (in elderly)
amnesia
dependence

Non-benzodiazepine hypnotics: diarrhoea, nausea and vomiting
vertigo and dizziness
headache
daytime drowsiness
depression
confusion
nightmares and perceptual disturbances
ataxia
bitter or metallic taste (zopiclone)

Residual effects

Ideally a hypnotic should only produce effects during the night, but this is not always the case and daytime sedation can be a problem. Residual effects include subjective feelings of sedation and objective impairment of psychomotor and cognitive function.

Residual effects seem to be most marked in normal volunteer subjects. All benzodiazepines impair speed of performance and reaction times, acquisition of new information and anterograde memory. Some tolerance does seem to develop when doses are repeated. In individuals with sleep disturbance the degree of impairment seems less (Bond & Lader 1996). Older people are particularly more likely to suffer adverse effects due to altered pharmacokinetics, especially in the elimination and metabolism of the longer acting benzodiazepine hypnotics. The newer non-benzodiazepines (zolpidem and zopiclone) are reported to produce less daytime sedation and cognitive impairment (Dujardin et al 1998) compared to benzodiazepines. Furthermore, zopiclone seems to have less deleterious effect on memory and cognitive function compared to zolpidem (Mattila et al 1998).

Rebound and withdrawal

Benzodiazepines typically reduce slow wave and REM sleep and prolong the time to the first REM episode. Thus a single dose of benzodiazepine supresses REM phase sleep but when the plasma concentration falls (that is during the following one or two nights) the amount of REM sleep is generally increased. This is called REM rebound. Following long-term administration, REM sleep does return to normal but abrupt withdrawal can lead to prolonged rebound which is often associated with intense dreams and anxiety on waking. This insomnia is usually worse than that experienced before commencement of the hypnotic and can lead to restarting of the hypnotic and possible dependence. Short-term administration and slow reduction in the night-time dose of the hypnotic over several days may reduce REM rebound. It is not yet clear if zopiclone and zolpidem have less rebound effect.

As described in Chapter 8, the cessation of benzodiazepines, even when used as hypnotics, can lead to withdrawal symptoms. The link between REM rebound and withdrawal symptoms remains unclear. The strategies employed to prevent withdrawal symptoms are the same as those used when benzodiazepines are prescribed as anxiolytics.

One important note: particularly in the UK, the illicit intravenous injection of temazepam has been a major problem. Marketed initially as a liquid-filled capsule, the contents could be injected easily. Even when marketed as gel-filled capsules, substance abusers found ways to liquify the gel for injection, but this tended to lead to major local tissue damage and gangrene, resulting in the loss of a limb in some cases. Consequently, additional controlled drug requirements have been applied to the prescribing of temazepam, and gel-filled preparations can no longer be prescribed within the National Health Service.

NON-PHARMACOLOGICAL INTERVENTIONS

It is now generally accepted that drugs used to promote sleep (hypnotics) should not be the first-line treatment for insomnia. Other, non-pharmacological, approaches such as cognitive therapy, autogenic training and stimulus control training should be explored. Morin et al (1993) examined the use of cognitive–behavioural therapy for late-life insomnia in adults over the age of 60 years. They stated that when medical causes are excluded, maladaptive behaviour and dysfunctional thoughts about sleep significantly affect older adults with sleep problems (Morin et al 1993). The combined cognitive and behavioural approach produced significantly positive objective and subjective ratings of sleep. Before therapy 54% of the subjects were taking regular sleeping medication but at 12-month follow-up no subject was taking regular medication (Morin et al 1993).

Mental health nurses and other health care professionals should perform an in-depth assessment and history of the nature of the sleep disturbance for each specific individual. Sleep problems should not be dismissed, and a complete assessment may highlight important aetiological factors. Furthermore, the assessment process may identify that the sleep expectation of an individual may be unrealistic or the impact and extent of alcohol consumption, which can cause insomnia, may not be recognised.

NARCOLEPSY

Narcolepsy is a disorder where excessive drowsiness is the main feature. Intense attacks of sleep, which last for between five and 30 minutes, occur at any time during the normal waking hours. Dantz et al (1994) describe narcolepsy as a disorder where uncontrolled attacks of sleep occur several times a day and usually last for 90 minutes. However, despite its prevalence of 0.03–0.05% of the population, narcolepsy is still often missed by health care professionals (Choo & Guilleminault 1998).

During a sleep attack, narcoleptics may lose muscle tone, a condition called cataplexy. As a result they may either experience weakness or be unable to maintain an upright position. Narcoleptics may also report sleep paralysis, which includes the temporary inability to move or talk while being conscious and aware of their surroundings, during which they may experience sensory hallucinations. Both sleep attacks and

---

Case study 9.3

Edward is a 36-year-old man who recently was suspended from work following an episode when he fell asleep at the wheel of his car while driving on the motorway. On initial questioning, Edward reported that he was often overcome with feelings of intense drowsiness, which would lead him to pull off the road and then he would fall asleep for periods lasting up to 30 minutes. Once he has had a sleep he feels refreshed and is able to continue with his work. These episodes occurred during the day but were unpredictable. He had been a heavy drinker in the past and for many years ascribed his drowsiness to the amount of alcohol he consumed. Edward did describe one time when he suddenly felt his limbs go weak and he collapsed and injured himself, although he remained conscious during this episode. He also reported waking up at night, being unable to move and having what he describes as waking dreams where he saw different things moving around in the bedroom that he knew the following morning were not really there. In retrospect he acknowledges that he has had a sleep problem for a long time in that he has tended to fall asleep inappropriately during most of his adult life.

A sleep EEG revealed reduced REM latency and typical features of narcolepsy. He was commenced on a low dosage of amphetamine. One year later he reported no further episodes of excessive drowsiness and he has been able to return to his job.

---

cataplexy may be precipitated by strong emotion, such as laughter or surprise.

Narcolepsy is an abnormality of REM sleep control, i.e. activity in the pons that produces REM sleep is not suppressed, so REM sleep occurs during usual wakeful hours (Hobson 1989). Indeed the duration and pattern of narcoleptic episodes are similar to the usual pattern of REM sleep.

Narcolepsy usually manifests between 15 and 25 years of age (Rosenzweig et al 1999), continues throughout life and is associated with significant psychosocial problems (Douglas 1998). No structural changes in the brain have been identified. Links with the human leucocyte antigen (HLA) system have been established and a specific HLA marker has been identified (Faraco et al 1999). Furthermore, in humans and animals narcolepsy is genetically inherited. In animals an autosomal recessive narcolepsy immune-related gene, named canarc-1, has been identified (Faraco et al 1999, Mignot et al 1993). This gene appears to be associated with increased acetylcholine receptor levels and release of acetylcholine in the pons reticular activating system (Aldrich 1993, Reid et al 1994).

Experimental findings suggest a hypersensitivity of the overall cholinergic system, which is linked to the limbic system, coupled with impaired dopamine release (Guilleminault et al 1998). The suggested link with the limbic system provides some explanation for the role of environmental factors in the provocation of narcoleptic episodes.

Narcolepsy requires long-term management. Interventions may be non-pharmacological, such as taking short naps at regular intervals, or pharmacological, involving the relief of daytime sleepiness by the use of CNS stimulants. Dexamphetamine has traditionally been used and recently modafinil has been introduced (Fry 1998), although dependence on modafinil with long-term use cannot be excluded and the recommendation is that it should be used with caution.

CONCLUSION

Sleep disorders are disabling for the individual as well as for carers. Various factors may account for short-term and transient sleep disturbance. Stress, anxiety, pain, increased environmental noise, changes in body temperature and dyspnoea, to name some, may all lead to poor sleep. However, changes in sleeping pattern may also be an early indicator of change in mood, including depression, particularly in elderly people. Health care professionals need to be committed to assessing sleep effectively and to be alert to changes in sleeping patterns. They should also develop the knowledge and skills to help individuals with sleep disorders to use, where appropriate, non-pharmacological strategies to restore good-quality sleep. Where pharmacological agents are used, health care professionals need to be alert for possible adverse effects and mindful of the possibility of psychological and physical dependence.

REFERENCES

Aidrich M A 1993 The neurobiology of nacrolepsy-cataplexy. Progress in Neurobiology 41: 533–541
Benca R M, Obermeyer W H, Thisted R A, Gillen J C 1992 Sleep and psychiatric disorders: a meta-analysis. Archives of General Psychiatry 49: 651–668
Bond A J, Lader M H 1996 Understanding drug treatment in mental health care. Wiley, Chichester
Bowersox S S, Kaitin K I, Dement W C 1985 EEG spindle activity as a function of age: relationship to sleep continuity. Brain Research 63: 526–539
Brabbins C J, Dewey M E, Copeland J R M et al 1993 Insomnia in the elderly: prevalence gender differences and relationships with morbidity and mortality. International Journal of Geriatric Psychiatry 10: 473–480
Carlson N R 1994 Physiology of behaviour, 5th edn. Allyn & Bacon, Boston
Choo K L, Guilleminault C 1998 Narcolepsy and idiopathic hypersomnolence. Clinics of Chest Medicine 19: 169–181
Dantz B, Edgar D M, Dement W C 1994 Circadian rhythms in narcolepsy: studies on a 90 minute day. Electroencephalography and Clinical Neurophysiology 90: 24–35
Douglas N J 1998 The psychosocial aspects of narcolepsy. Neurology 50(2 suppl 1): S27–S30
Dujardin K, Guieu J D, Leconte-Lambert C, Leconte P, Borderies P, de La Giclais B 1998 Comparison of the effects of zolpidem and flunitrazepam on sleep structure and daytime cognitive functions. A study of untreated insomniacs. Pharmacopsychiatry 31: 14–18
Faraco J, Lin X, Li R, Hinton L, Lin L, Mignot E 1999 Genetic studies in narcolepsy: a disorder affecting REM sleep. Journal of Heredity 90: 129–132
Fry J M 1998 Treatment modalities for narcolepsy. Neurology 50(2 suppl 1): S43–S48

Guilleminault C, Heinzer R, Mignot E, Black J 1998 Investigations into the neurologic basis of narcolepsy. Neurology 50(2 suppl 1): S8–S15

Halasz P, Pal I, Rajna P 1985 K complex formation of the EEG in sleep: a survey and new examinations. Acta Physiologica Hungaria 65: 3–35

Hobson J A 1989 Sleep. Scientific American Library, New York

Horne J A 1988 Why we sleep: the functions of sleep in humans and other mammals. Oxford University Press, Oxford

Lancel, M (1999) Role of GABA$_A$ receptors in the regulation of sleep: initial sleep responses to peripherally administered modulators and agonists. Sleep 22: 33–42

Leonard B E 1992 Fundamentals of psychopharmacology. Wiley, Chichester

McGinty D, Szymusiak R 1990 Keeping cool: a hypothesis about the mechanisms and function of slow-wave sleep. Trends in Neurosciences 13: 480–487

Mattila M J, Vanakoski J, Kalska H, Seppala T 1998 Effects of alcohol, zolpidem and some other sedatives and hypnotics on human performance and memory. Pharmacology, Biochemistry and Behaviour 59: 917–923

Mignot E, Nishino S, Sharp L H et al 1993 Heterozygosity at the canarc-1 locus can confer susceptibility for narcolepsy: induction of cataplexy in heterozygous asymptomatic dogs after administration of a combination of drugs acting on monoaminergic and cholinergic systems. Journal of Neuroscience 13: 1057–1064

Morin C M, Kowatch R A, Barry T, Walton E 1993 Cognitive–behaviour therapy for late-life insomnia. Journal of Consulting and Clinical Psychology 61: 137–146

Oswald I 1987 The benefit of sleep. Holistic Medicine 2: 137–139

Reid M S, Tafti M, Nishino C, Siegel J M, Dement W C, Mignot E 1994 Cholinergic regulation of cataplexy in canine narcolepsy in the pontine reticular formation is mediated by M$_2$ mucscarinic receptors. Sleep 17: 424–435

Rosenzweig M R, Leiman A L, Breedlove S M 1999 Biological psychology: an introduction to behavioural, cognitive and clinical neuroscience. Sinauer, Massachusetts

Shapiro C M, Dement W C 1993 Impact and epidemiology of sleep disorders. British Medical Journal 306: 1604–1607

Smith C 1985 Sleep states and learning: a review of the animal literature. Neuroscience and Biobehavioural Reviews 9: 157–168

Smith C, Lapp L 1991 Increased number of REMs following an intensive learning experience in college students. Sleep Research 14: 325–330

Thase M E 1998 Depression, sleep and antidepressants. Journal of Clinical Psychiatry 59 (suppl 4): 55–65

Trimble M R 1996 Biological psychiatry, 2nd edn. Wiley, Chichester

Vanderwolf C H 1992 The electrocardiogram in relation to physiology and behaviour: a new analysis. Electroencephalography and Clinical Neurophysiology 82: 165–175

10

Stress, the individual and mental health

Only when an event is perceived by a human being, evaluated and appraised as dangerous, or a threat to self-esteem or loss of personal resources, does the stressor elicit distress.

(Millenson, 1995)

Key Points

- Stress is the totality of disruption to homeostasis by a stimulus coupled with the response by the individual
- The perception an individual has about an event or object makes it a stressor
- There is a neuroendocrine response to stress or stressors
- The primary response to most stressful situations is via the catecholaminergic and hypothalamo-pituitary-adrenal (HPA) axis
- Higher natural killer (NK) cell activity is a marker for the ability to cope with life event stressors

---

The concept of stress is one that is most researched in the field of psychophysiology. Although there is a proliferation of literature on stress and many people have attempted to define stress, no one has been able to produce a definition of stress that is acceptable to most people. Selye (1956) defined stress in two different ways: one views stress as the rate of wear and tear within the body; the other describes stress as the state manifested by a specific syndrome which consists of all the non-specifically induced changes within a biological system.

Millenson (1995) gives a very brief but interesting summary and analysis of Selye's work and findings in mice and the complexities that have been experienced when some of these studies are extended to the human species. While physicists and psychobiologists infer different meanings of stress, as Millenson (1995) explains very clearly, the notion of some 'force' or 'forces' or 'stressors' is implicit in the word stress. Indeed the Concise Oxford Dictionary (Sykes 1976) defines stress as 'a constraining or impelling force' and as 'an effort or demand upon physical or mental energy'. Another definition worth considering is that given by Murray & Huelskoetter (1991, p 333) who define stress as:

a physical and emotional state always present in the person as a result of living; it is intensified in a non-specific response to an internal or external environmental change or threat. It is a dynamic state of imbalance in response to demands, threats, challenges, unmet needs, or lack of resources. The body's non-specific response to being stressed is always the same, although in the stress reaction, the body also manifests a reaction specific to each agent.

The length of the latter definition sums up how difficult it is to define stress. This chapter explores the notion of stressors in human existence and the nature of the mind–body response to such stressors. Aspects of the demand upon physical or mental energy or both are discussed and the possible pathways that lead to physical and mental fatigue are examined coupled with the physiological and psychological adaptations (or lack of such adaptations) to stressors and fatigue.

Burgess (1997) defines stress in two different ways: (1) stress is a stimulus that upsets an individual's balance or homeostasis; and (2) stress is an individual's response to a stressful stimulus. In this chapter we define stress as the totality of the disruption to the individual's homeostasis by a stimulus or stimuli coupled with the general and specific response by

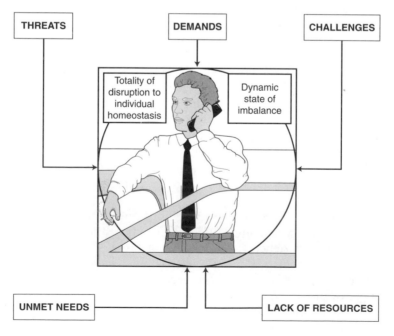

Figure 10.1 Stress as the totality of disruption to individual homeostasis.

the individual. The factors that cause this totality of disruption are shown in Figure 10.1.

THE BIOPSYCHOSOCIAL ASPECTS OF STRESS

An impossible question to answer completely but worth asking is: what are the human stressors? Many stressors are what can be described as the shared life experience of humankind that many people encounter on the life continuum. An illustration of the potential stressors in human existence is given in Figure 10.2. Such an illustration causes problems since many of the stressors can fit into several categories, but it still serves as a useful reminder.

A different but challenging classification of stressors has been put forward by Millenson (1995). He groups the various types of stressors into:

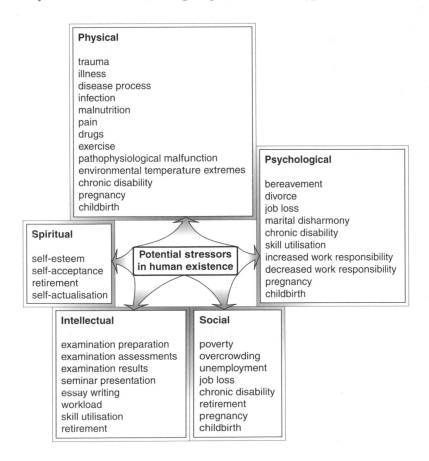

Figure 10.2   Potential stressors in human existence.

Table 10.1 Classification of stressors

Type of stressor	Example of situation, event
Acute (time-limited)	Visit to dentist, physical injury, awaiting medical investigation results
Sequential	Marriage, pregnancy, childbirth, divorce, bereavement, job loss
Chronic intermittent	Examination preparation, examination assessments, essay writing, production deadlines, high-powered meetings
Chronic ongoing	Debilitating illness, long-term exposure to occupational hazards, long-term relationship disharmony, absolute poverty, mundane tasks, difficult employer, academic pressure

acute (time-limited), such as a visit to the dentist, a driving test, awaiting results of a medical test; sequential, such as marriage, divorce and bereavement; chronic intermittent, such as examinations and deadlines; and, finally, chronic ongoing, such as debilitating illness, poverty, long-term exposure to environmental or occupational hazards and prolonged relationship discord. Table 10.1 shows an adaptation of Millenson's classification of stressors. What is apparent in this grouping is not only the nature of the stressor but also its intensity and the time factor involved, or how long the stressor is experienced by the recipient.

So what makes an event or situation a stressor? Epictetus (c 60AD–100AD, Russell 1989) one of the stoic philosophers stated, 'men are disturbed not by things but by the views they take of them' (Millenson 1995). Thus it is the *perception an individual has* about an event or object that makes it a stressor. A different viewpoint, a mundane task, an uttered phrase, the colour of another person (and hence racism), a desired lifestyle can all be stressors to different people, while at the same time none of these could be stressors for others. Indeed, as one observes and ponders about the hustle and bustle of city life and modern living coupled with biopsychosocial complexities that are experienced by people of all ages, including young people maturing early, one is bound to conclude that there are so many people so busy trying to get somewhere that they never have the time to enjoy what they have.

In a series of experiments in animals and in humans, Seligman (1975) showed that if successful coping is denied or where access to coping behaviour is not available for whatever reason, exposure to stressful situations leads to behaviour breakdown, which he termed 'learned helplessness'. It is not the authors' intention to discuss learned helplessness in this chapter as many psychology textbooks and papers do justice to this term and discuss it in detail (Abrahamson et al 1980, Rungapadiacy 1999, Seligman 1975). Seligman's work is well discussed by Rungapadiacy (1999) who states that when an organism experiences trauma that it cannot control, it shows waning motivation to respond to later trauma. The point to make here that is linked with learned helplessness is that when attempts to cope with the stressors cease, there is lack of adaptation or breakdown in adaptation to the stress. Associated with the issue of adaptation is the perception that individuals have about the focus of control in their lives and health (Cullen 1984). Scales that measure the locus of control are discussed by Rotter (1966, 1975), Wallston et al (1978) and Wallston & Wallston (1981). The locus of control scales or measures seek to identify whether individuals perceive the influence on their lives to be within their control or whether this control is by others or external events. It can be deduced from this that there is no doubt that more stressors are experienced where individuals perceive the locus of control on their lives to be external or to be with others.

Whether an encounter, situation or event will produce challenge or threat appraisals has been discussed by Averill (1973), Lefcourt (1976) and Lazarus & Folkman (1984) and very much depends on the extent to which people feel confident of their powers of mastery over the environment or, alternatively, feel great vulnerability to harm in a world conceived as dangerous and hostile.

Since a significant percentage of the world population spend their life working for a living, one useful category to explore briefly is that of occupational stressors and where the locus of control lies. Previous studies have explored various aspects of occupational stressors. Theorell (1974) found that there was a significant association between occupational life changes and the incidence of myocardial infarction, and reports his patients citing factors that include: change to a different line of work; decreased or increased responsibility; major change in work schedule; trouble with colleagues or with the boss; and retirement from work. All these factors signify some shift in the locus of control. Theorell's work is supported by Marmot et al (1978) who also found significant correlation between occupational grade and coronary heart disease among British civil servants. Other studies have focused on the stresses of 'blue-collar' (Poulton 1978) and 'white-collar' workers (Cooper & Marshall 1978).

Lazarus & Folkman (1984) cite studies by Vogel et al (1959) that support the view that vulnerability to stress (especially psychological stress) is very much related to commitment. Indeed Lazarus & Folkman (1984) state that the greater the strength of a commitment, the more vulnerable the person is to psychological stress in the area of that commitment.

Another important concept to understand that is related to stress is that of cognitive appraisal. Cognitive appraisal refers to evaluative cognitive processes that intervene between the encounter of the stressor and the reaction (Lazarus & Folkman 1984). They argue that individuals are able to evaluate the significance of what is happening to their well-being through cognitive appraisal processes. Thus commitment influences cognitive appraisal by guiding individuals into and away from situations that can challenge and benefit them on one hand or threaten and harm them on the other (Lazarus & Folkman 1984).

Steptoe (1991) argues that in addition to contributing to the onset of illness, psychosocial factors are also significant in that they affect the course, severity and prognosis of a condition. Hobbis (1996) describes the mediating psychological variables that may have a beneficial effect and are available to the individual as psychosocial resources. These resources moderate the effects of a stressor and include prior experience of the stressor, the wider social context of the individual and the personality traits or characteristics of the individual.

Optimism (Sarafino 1994) and 'hardiness' (Kobasa 1979, Kobasa et al 1982) are two significant personality traits believed to moderate effects of stressors. The same authors conclude from their studies that the three factors that constitute 'hardiness' are control, commitment and challenge and that all three factors work in an interrelated fashion to protect the individual from the adverse effects of stress. However, Lazarus & Folkman (1984) question the sensitivity of the tools (personality scales) used to measure hardiness by Kobasa and colleagues (1979, 1982) and wonder whether the tools used were measuring issues of alienation and security.

NEUROENDOCRINE INTERACTION AS A STRESS RESPONSE

It is possible that the neuroendocrine responses to stress or stressors has an evolutionary link since the nervous and endocrine systems interact with and complement each other. Anatomically the vertebrate pituitary gland has evolved as a fusion between neural tissue and epithelial tissue and is very closely linked to the hypothalamus, by the hypothalamo-pituitary stalk. Functionally the nervous system has a regulatory effect on the pituitary via the hypothalamus and the pituitary itself is also influenced by feedback mechanisms from the secretions of other endocrine glands (Daggett 1981, Hardy 1984).

Activation of the hypothalamo-pituitary-adrenal (HPA) axis is part of the physiological response to stress. Adrenocorticotrophic hormone (ACTH) produced by the anterior pituitary gland stimulates production of cortisol and corticosterone by the adrenal cortex, the outside portion of the suprarenal glands that lie on top of the kidneys. During brief stressful situations, the autonomic nervous system (ANS) stimulates the adrenal medulla to increase its secretion of adrenaline. Psychophysiological studies with Swedish male high school students whose accomplishments were greater than their intelligence scores (overachievers) showed that they secreted more adrenaline (epinephrine) in an achievement-demanding situation than other boys in the same class. These findings have been interpreted to mean that subjects predominately orientated to achievement are more disturbed by achievement-related stimuli whereas those more orientated to affiliation are more disturbed by affiliation threat (Lazarus & Folkman 1984). However, if the stressful situation persists, the adrenal cortex is involved via the hypothalamus and pituitary gland. Chronic stress may cause severe illness and even death. Both cortisol and corticosterone promote the formation of glucose in the liver (a process known as gluconeogenesis) and thus help in maintaining normal blood sugar levels. For this reason cortisol and corticosterone are known as glucocorticoid hormones.

James (1884) concluded from his studies of perceiving and brain function that emotions are perceptions of changes within the body itself. James (1884) argued that people's emotional feelings are based on what they find themselves doing as well as on the sensory feedback they receive from the activity of their muscles and internal organs. This means that individuals self-observe where emotional feelings are concerned and when individuals find themselves uneasy and trembling, they experience fear. This theory was supported by Lange (1887), a Danish physiologist and became known as the James–Lange theory (Hilgard et al 1979). Carlson (1998) summarises the James–Lange theory as a theory of emotion that suggests that behaviours and physiological responses are elicited directly by situations and that feelings of emotions are produced by feedback from these behaviours and responses.

Further clarification of the structure and function of the ANS contributed to the study of visceral correlates of subjective emotional states. This led Cannon (1914) to draw attention to the close relationships between emotional activity and sympathetic function and to his emergency theory of emotion which stated that the sympathetic division of the autonomic nervous system helps the organism to face stress. Furthermore, he suggested that all the symptoms of sympathetic activation increase resistance to stress and enhance defensive abilities (the fight-or-flight reaction). The sympathetic nervous system produces a whole body response during emergencies and sudden environmental changes. This ability is an important part by which individuals respond to stressors. Any stressful situation leading to rage or fear may result in increased cardiac output, heart rate, blood pressure, blood sugar, respiration and perspiration. However, later studies and anecdotal evidence (Hohman 1966, Sweet 1966 cited in Carlson 1998), while supporting Cannon's findings, do show the importance of feedback mechanisms from other parts of the body to the brain and the characteristic combinations of sympathetic and parasympathetic effects, as shown by the defaecation and urination experienced by frightened soldiers, both processes of which are under parasympathetic control. In this case, fear is the stressor.

Cannon (1927) opposed the James–Lange theory and together with Bard's contribution proposed the Cannon–Bard theory a few years later. Cannon argued that the internal organs were not sensitive enough to produce feedback that could account for emotional feelings by individuals. But as Carlson (1998) explains, later research finds Cannon and Bard's criticisms unfounded or invalid since some changes within the viscera do occur quickly enough to cause feelings of emotion.

THE UNIFIED STRESS MODEL

The definition we have given in this chapter focusing on the totality of the disruption to the individual's homeostasis and the response by the individual has inherent properties of a unified stress model. It encompasses not only the potential stressors in human existence as stimuli

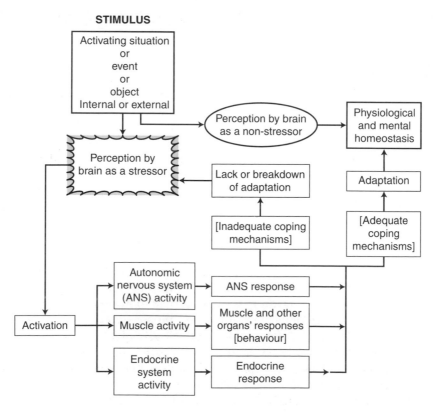

Figure 10.3 The Rinomhota–Marshall stress model. Adapted from Carlson (1998). A diagrammatic representation of the James– theory of emotion.

but also the coping mechanisms within the individual, issues of perception, aspects of locus of control and adaptation. Figure 10.3 shows this unified stress model whereby both the short- and long-term effects of stress are seen. In this unified model, any of the five dimensions of the individual (physical, emotional, intellectual, social and spiritual) has potential to or can generate a situation or event (the stimulus) that can be perceived by the brain as a stressor and, in addition, the nature of the mind–body response to the stressor, coping mechanisms inherent in the individual and how the individual adapts are all illustrated. It must be emphasised here that adaptation is a continuation of the initial ANS, endocrine, muscle and other organ responses. Adequate coping mechanisms to the activating stimulus lead to quick adaptation and a restoration of homeostasis. However, inadequate coping mechanisms lead to lack of or breakdown in adaptation and a cycle of chronic stress with the possibility of the development of mental illness.

STRESS, CHRONIC FATIGUE SYNDROME AND THE IMMUNE RESPONSE

In chapter 6 the link between chronic fatigue syndrome (CFS) and immune function was discussed. Demitrack (1994) suggested that hormonal dysfunction centred around the HPA axis may be responsible for CFS. The unifying approach by Krupp & Pollina (1996), in which elevated stress and poor coping skills having an effect on immune function, leading to CFS and prolonged illness, links well with other issues of locus of control, vulnerability to harm, inherent coping mechanisms and adaptation that have been discussed earlier in this chapter.

There is abundant evidence to support the view that physical illness is stressful to the body and to the individual and eventually leads to fatigue. Fatigue has been demonstrated in rheumatoid arthritis (Belza et al 1993), in systemic lupus erythematosus (Hastings et al 1986, Krupp et al 1990), in Parkinson's disease (Friedman & Friedman 1993, Van Hilten et al 1993), in multiple sclerosis (Freal et al 1984) and in HIV (Darko et al 1992), to mention but a few. Individuals suffering from cancer experience severe and disabling fatigue due to the chemotherapy and radiotherapy they undergo. On their reviews on cancer and fatigue, Aistars (1987) and Smets et al (1993) have placed great emphasis on the multifactorial nature of the problem and cite anaemia, depression, drugs, immobilisation and malnutrition as all having some contribution to the fatigue. The stress–fatigue relationship is shown in Figure 10.4.

Fatigue in physical illness has been found in many studies to correlate with psychological factors. In particular, fatigue correlates with ratings of depression (Friedman & Friedman 1993, McKinley et al 1995), poor

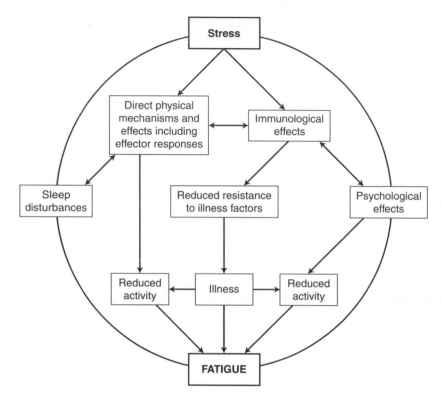

Figure 10.4 Stress-fatigue relationship. Adapted from Wessely et al 1998 by permission of Oxford University Press.

sleep, functional disability, depressive symptoms and low haematocrit (Belza 1995), and pain, depression and duration of illness (Blesch et al 1991). The issue of fatigue and emotional disorders especially depression and anxiety has been reviewed more recently by Wessely et al (1998).

Earlier Aistars (1987) had postulated that psychological factors lead to chronic fatigue and labelled anxiety, depression and crisis as energy-depleting states. Aistars (1987) also proposed a theoretical model linking the reticular activating system (RAS) with fatigue. The RAS is located in the reticular formation of the midbrain and medulla and is responsible for maintaining wakefulness and alerting the cortex. Astairs argues that fatigue is an outward manifestation of the RAS being inhibited. This occurs as a result of lowered sensory input, decreased response to input that includes sensory deprivation, immobility and isolation, and reduced cortical activity through chronic stimulation such as anxiety, depression, narcotics and pain. Claus et al (1996) support this theoretical model but argue that it is difficult to separate the cognitive and affective elements within it. Other studies (Risdale et al 1994) also show correlation between fatigue and emotional distress, while Komaroff (1993) supported the link between fatigue and depression and stated that among all patients who seek medical care for fatigue, depression (with or without associated anxiety disorders or somatization) is by far the most common cause. Mumford (1994) also concluded that fatigue and weakness are more closely associated with depressive disorder than any other psychiatric diagnosis even though this is not specific. However, the conclusion reached by other workers (Fuhrer & Wessely 1995, Hawton et al 1990) is that while there is an association between depression and fatigue, there is also a similar association between fatigue and non-psychiatric diagnosis and hence fatigue is not a discriminating symptom for depression.

Wessely et al (1998) cite Hemphill et al (1952) as stating that fatigue is part and parcel of our concepts of anxiety. Clinical studies by Winokur & Holeman (1963), Angst & Dobler Milola (1985), Buchwald et al (1987) and Kroenke et al (1988) show the link between anxiety disorders and chronic fatigue. In particular, symptoms that included weakness, exhaustion, poor concentration, hypersensitivity and substantial fatigue were very common in those with anxiety disorder (Angst & Dobler Milola 1985). Although the sample sizes were small, Kiecolt-Glaser and fellow workers (1987) found that separated or divorced women had a poorer immune function on five of six immunological variables studied than matched married women while Kiecolt-Glaser & Glaser (1988) reported similar findings in separated or divorced men. In a prospective longitudinal study of spouses of women with advanced breast cancer, Schleifer et al (1983) noticed that mitogen-stimulated lymphocyte response in the spouses was significantly lower during the first two months following the death of their wives when compared to the period before death. They also noticed that in the majority of cases, this lymphocyte response was normal a year after the death of the wife. An earlier study by Clayton et al (1972) had found depressed mood in bereaved subjects, and the same authors inferred a causal relationship between stress-induced depression and abnormal lymphocyte function.

Using natural killer (NK) cell activity as a marker for the ability to cope, Locke and co-workers (1984) examined the effects of cell-mediated immunity in a group of undergraduate student volunteers and their findings show that those individuals with an ability to cope with life event stressors had significantly higher NK cell activity than those less able to cope with the stressors. They also found that there was an inverse relationship between NK cell activity and psychiatric symptoms of anxiety and depression. They concluded that anxiety and depression may have a negative effect on immune function.

Both examination stress and academic stress in medical students have been reported to cause significant changes in antibody titre in response to herpes simplex virus, Epstein-Barr virus and cytomegalovirus, thus suggesting changes in immunity (Glaser et al 1986, Kiecolt-Glaser & Glaser 1991, Kiecolt-Glaser et al 1984, Leonard 1995). In these studies there was decreased NK cell activity and increased titres of antibodies. Leonard (1995) concludes that although there are well-established adaptive effects of severe experimentally induced psychological stress in animals on immunocompetence, the effects of adverse life events and stress in humans may not produce similarly pronounced adaptive changes. Certainly as Leonard (1995) points out, there are many studies that support the view that there is a relationship between stressors and immune defences but there still remains the problem of deciding which parameters reflect, with accuracy, the true status of the individual's immune response to stressors.

Case study 10.1

Julie is a 49-year-old woman who has worked as a primary school teacher for over 20 years. For the past 12 years she has worked in the same primary school and over most of this time has coped well with her responsibilities. She has always been an extremely conscientious woman who was liked by her pupils and also by their parents. Over the years she has has been a member of the school governing body and over the past six years has adopted the role of specialist needs coordinator. Four years ago a new headmistress was appointed to the school who then appointed Julie formally as a special needs coordinator in addition to her responsibilities as a class teacher and in different out-of-school activities with different children.

Julie's husband recently took early retirement due to physical ill health. Her mother is in a nursing home and suffers from dementia. Julie has now been off sick from work for the past six months and is applying for medical retirement. She is surprised to report that she was under stress over four years previously when in retrospect she realises that her sleep was disturbed, as she would wake up in the early hours each morning worrying about preparation for school the following day. She also realises that she was working seven days a week during term time and taking work preparation through into the holiday periods. She was aware that her concentration had declined; she was rather sharper with her pupils and less understanding. During the two weeks prior to being seen by her family doctor and a psychiatrist, Julie had become more depressed in her mood, increasingly sleepless, more anxious and panicky in class. Julie continued to struggle on although a number of her colleagues commented on how ill she looked. Things came to a head as she was preparing class reports and reports for a special needs function of her job for an Ofsted inspection. Although she coped well during the week of the Ofsted visit, the following week she collapsed, became extremely tearful, was unable to face the children in class and went off sick. She has not returned to her job since that time.

Over the past five months she has become fearful of receiving any phone calls, has been avoiding going near the school and cannot watch television if there is any mention of teaching or school. She actively avoids her former pupils or parents and feels guilty about being unable to cope with the demands of her job. When contacted by the school about the future, she becomes acutely panic-stricken and passes the handling of these problems to her husband.

THE GENERAL ADAPTATION SYNDROME

The general adaptation syndrome is a way the body reacts or responds to stress and was first described by Selye (1956). Since many authors have reviewed this syndrome, it will suffice in this text to mention that the three phases of the general adaptation syndrome include the alarm phase, the adaptation phase and exhaustion. More recent reviews have been given by Murray & Huelskoetter (1991), Millenson (1995) and Rungapadiacy (1999).

The Alarm Phase

The alarm phase is a typical fight-or-flight reaction which is an immediate, short-term, life-preserving sympathetic nervous system response to a stressor. The perception of a stressor triggers release of corticotrophin hormone releasing factor (CRF) which influences the hypothalamus to produce other hormones that initiate a cascade of physiological responses. These responses include: dilation of pupils; increased cardiac rate, strength and output; increased blood flow to brain, heart and skeletal muscles; tension in head and shoulder muscles leading to headaches; dilation of bronchi with increased muscle tone; increased cellular metabolism; breakdown of fat to form free fatty acids that can be used by muscles; synthesis of more glucose from glycerol; increased ADH and aldosterone production; retention of salt and water by kidneys in order to boost blood volume; and breakdown of glycogen to make more glucose.

The Resistance Phase

The resistance phase is an adaptation stage that occurs due to continued exposure to the stressor or threat and is the body's way of adapting to the instability caused by the stressors. Neuroendocrine responses such as adrenocortical responses facilitate changes that enable the body to fight for self-preservation. This involves anabolic reactions and mobilisation of all the body's resources. It is highly likely that the variables of psychosocial resources, optimism and 'hardiness' discussed earlier in this chapter are part of this resistance or adaptation phase and help to define the individual differences in the ability to cope with stress.

Exhaustion

The phase of exhaustion results from long-term continued exposure to stressors from both the internal and the external environments coupled with inadequate adaptive mechanisms. It is in this phase when resources are depleted that irreversible damage to tissues or to the individual occurs and this is sometimes followed by illness and death (Murray & Huelskoetter 1991).

CONCLUSION

Whatever the specificity and non-specificity of issues surrounding stress, there is no doubt that the primary response in most stressful situations in both humans and animals involves the catecholaminergic and HPA axis. The principal players are the brain, the sympathetic nervous system, the adrenal medulla and the HPA axis.

There is an immunosuppressive effect of stress in both humans and animals (Ader & Cohen 1993, Kiecolt-Glaser & Glaser 1991). Many human experiences show that when individuals are under acute stress situations such as an examination, an impending infection can be delayed until when the pressure is relieved, a point at which immunological resistance collapses suddenly. Thus, activation of the immune system is correlated with altered neurophysiological, neurochemical and neuroendocrine activities in the brain (Leonard 1995).

From a biopsychosocial perspective, it can be argued that coping mechanisms encompass physiological processes, cognitive strategies such as appraisal and use of psychosocial resources in order to produce adaptation. De Ridder & Schreurs (1996) add that an individual's ability to appraise the degree of threat from any stressor is very much influenced by the attitudes, beliefs and expectations that the individual has about the given situation. Thus, individuals respond to stressors at physiological, psychological and behavioural levels.

REFERENCES

Abrahamson L Y, Garber J, Seligman M E P 1980 Learned helplessness in humans: an attributional analysis. In: Garber J, Seligman M E P (eds) Human helplessness, theory and applications. Academic Press, New York
Ader R, Cohen N 1993 Psychoneuroimmunology: conditioning and stress. Annual Review of Psychology 44: 53–85
Aistars J 1987 Fatigue in the cancer patient: a conceptual approach to a clinical problem. Oncology Nursing Forum 14: 25–30
Angst J, Dobler Milola A 1985 The Zurich study v anxiety and phobia in young adults. European Archives of Psychiatry and Neurological Sciences 235(3): 171–178
Averill J R 1973 Personal control over aversive stimuli and its relationship to stress. Psychological Bulletin 80: 286–303
Belza B L 1995 Comparison of self report fatigue in rheumatoid arthritis and controls. Journal of Rheumatology 22: 639–643

Belza B L, Henke C J, Yelin E H, Epstein W V, Gilliss C L 1993 Correlates of fatigue in older adults with rheumatoid arthritis. Nursing Research 42: 93–99

Blesch K S, Paice J A, Wickham R et al 1991 Correlates of fatigue in people with breast or lung cancer. Oncology Nursing Forum 18: 81–87

Buchwald D, Sullivan J, Komaroff A 1987 Frequency of chronic active Epstein-Barr virus infection in a general medical practice. Journal of the American Medical Association 257: 2303–2307

Burgess A W 1997 Psychiatric nursing – promoting mental health. Appleton & Lange, London

Cannon W B 1914 The emergency function of the adrenal medulla in pain and major emotions. American Journal of Physiology 33: 356–372

Cannon W B 1927 The James-Lange theory of emotions: a critical examination and an alternative. American Journal of Psychology 39: 106–124

Carlson N R 1998 Physiology of behaviour, 6th edn. Allyn & Bacon, Boston

Claus A, Crow R, Hammond S 1996 A qualitative study to explore the concept of fatigue/tiredness in cancer patients and in healthy individuals. European Journal of Cancer Care 5(suppl 2): 8–23

Clayton P J, Halikes J A, Maurice W L 1972 The depression of widowhood. British Journal of Psychiatry 120: 71–80

Cooper C L, Marshall J 1978 Sources of managerial and white collar stress. In: Cooper C L, Payne R (eds) Stress at work. Wiley, Chichester, p 81–105

Cullen J 1984 Towards a taxonomy of methods – a general overview of psychological approaches in the study of breakdown of human adaptation. In: Cullen J, Siegrist J (eds) Breakdown in human adaptation to stress – towards a nultidisciplinary approach, vol 1, part 1. Martinus Nijhoff, Boston, p 3–37

Daggett P 1981 Clinical endocrinology. Edward Arnold, London

Darko D F, McCutchan J A, Kripke D F, Gillian J C, Golshan S 1992 Fatigue, sleep disturbance, disability and indices of progression of HIV infection. American Journal of Psychiatry 149: 514–520

Demitrack M A 1994 Chronic fatigue syndrome: a disease of the hypothalamic–pituitary – adrenal axis? Annals of Medicine 26: 1–5

De Ridder D, Schreurs K 1996 Coping, social support and chronic disease: a research agenda. Psychology, Health and Medicine 1(1): 71–82

Freal J E, Kraft G H, Coryell J K 1984 Symptomatic fatigue in multiple sclerosis. Archives of Physical Medicine and Rehabilitation 65: 135–138

Friedman J, Friedham H 1993 Fatigue in Parkinson's disease. Neurology 43: 2016–2019

Fuhrer R, Wessely S 1995 Fatigue in French primary care. Psychological Medicine 25: 895–905

Glaser R, Rice T, Speicher C E, Stout J C, Kiecolt-Glaser J K 1986 Stress depresses interferon production by leucocytes concomitant with a decrease in natural killer cell activity. Behavioral Neuroscience 100: 675–678

Hardy R N 1984 Endocrine Physiology. Edward Arnold, London

Hastings C, Joyce K, Yarboro C, Berkebile C, Yocum D 1986 Factors affecting fatigue in systemic lupus erythematosus. Arthritis and Rheumatism 29 (suppl): 5176

Hawton K, Mayou R, Feldman E 1990 Significance of psychiatric symptoms in general medical patients with mood disorders. General Hospital Psychiatry 12: 296–302

Hemphill R, Hall K, Crookes T 1952 A preliminary report on fatigue and pain tolerance in depressive and psychoneurotic patients. Journal of Mental Science 98: 433–440

Hilgard E R, Atkinson R L, Atkinson R C 1979 Introduction to psychology, 7th edn. Harcourt Brace, New York

Hobbis I 1996 Significance of psychological and psychosocial variables in the presentation of chronic idiopathic constipation. PhD thesis, University of Sheffield

Hohman C W 1966 Some effects of spinal cord lesions on experienced emotional feelings. Psychophysiology 3: 143–156

James W 1884 What is an emotion? Mind 9: 188–205

Kiecolt-Glaser J K, Glaser R 1988 Methodological issues in behavioural immunology research in humans. Brain Behaviour and Immunology 2: 67–78

Kiecolt-Glaser J K, Glaser R 1991 Stress and immune functions in humans. In Ader R, Fetten D L, Cohen N (eds) Psychoneuroimmunology. Academic Press, San Diego, p 849–867

Kiecolt-Glaser J K, Garner W, Speicher C E, Penn G, Glaser R 1984 Psychosocial modifiers of immunocompetence in medical students. Psychosomatic Medicine 46: 7–14

Kiecolt-Glaser T K, Fisher L, Ogrockie P, Stout J C, Speicher C E, Glaser R 1987 Methodological issues in behavioural immunology research in humans. Brain Behaviour and Immunology 2: 67–78

Kobasa S C 1979 Stressful life events, personality and health – an inquiry into hardiness. Journal of Personality and Social Psychology 37: 1–11

Kobasa S C, Maddi S R, Kahn S 1982 Hardiness and health: prospective study. Journal of Personality and Social Psychology 42: 168–177

Komaroff A 1993 Clinical presentation of chronic fatigue syndrome. In: Brock G R, Whelan J (eds) Chronic fatigue syndrome. Wiley, Chichester, p 43–61

Kroenke K, Wood D, Mangelsdorff D, Meier N, Powell J 1988 Chronic fatigue in primary care: prevalence, patient characteristics and outcome. Journal of the American Medical Association 260: 929–934

Krupp L B, Pollina D 1996 Neuroimmune and neuropsychiatric aspects of chronic fatigue syndrome. Advances in Neuroimmunology 6: 155–167

Lazarus R S, Folkman S 1984 Stress, appraisal and coping. Springer, New York

Lefcourt H M 1976 Locus of control: current trends in theory and research. Halstead, New York

Leonard B E 1995 Stress and the immune system: immunological aspects of depressive illness. In: Leonard B E, Miller K (eds) Stress, the immune system and psychiatry. Wiley, Chichester, p 113–136

Locke S E, Kraus L, Leserman J 1984 Life change, stress, psychiatric symptoms and natural killer-cell activity. Psychosomatic Medicine 46: 441–453

McKinley P S, Ouellette S C, Winkel G H 1995 The contributions of disease activity, sleep patterns and depression to fatigue in systemic lupus erythematosus. Arthritis and Rheumatology 38: 826–834

Marmot M G, Rose G, Shipley M, Hamilton P J S 1978 Employment grade and coronary heart disease in British civil servants. Journal of Epidemiology and Community Health 32: 244–252

Millenson J R 1995 Mind matters – psychosocial medicine in holistic practice. Eastlands Press, Seattle

Mumford D 1994 Can 'functional' somatic symptoms associated with anxiety and depression be differentiated? International Journal in Methodology and Psychological Research 4: 133–141

Murray R B, Huelskoetter M M W 1991 The person on the health–illness continuum: promoting adaptation to the stress response. In: Murray R B, Huelskoetter M M W (eds) Psychiatric mental health nursing – giving emotional care, 3rd edn. Appleton & Lange, Norwalk, p 329–388

Poulton E C 1978 Blue collar stressors. In: Cooper C L, Payne R (eds) Stress at work. Wiley, Chichester, p 51–79

Ridsdale L, Evans A, Jerrett W, Mandalia S, Ostler K, Vora H 1994 Patients who consult with tiredness: frequency of consultation, perceived causes of tiredness and its association with psychological distress. British Journal of General Practice 44: 413–416

Rotter J B 1966 Generalised expectancies for internal versus external control of reinforcement. Psychological Monographs 80(1): 1–28

Rotter J B 1975 Some problems and misconceptions related to the construct of internal versus external control of reinforcement. Journal of Consulting and Clinical Psychology 43: 56–67

Rungapadiacy D M 1999 Interpersonal communication and psychology for health care professionals–theory and practice. Butterworth-Heinemann, Oxford

Russell B 1989 Wisdom of the west. Bloomsbury, London, p 112

Sarafino E P 1994 Health psychology: biopsychosocial interactions, 2nd edn. Wiley, Chichester

Schleifer S J, Keller S E, Camerimi M, Thornton C J, Stein M 1983 Suppression of lymphocyte stimulation following bereavement. Journal of the American Medical Association 250: 374–377

Seligman M E P 1975 Helplessness. W H Freeman, San Francisco

Selye H 1956 The stress of life. Reprint (reviewed edition) 1990 McGraw-Hill, New York

Smets E M A, Garssen B, Shuster-Uitterhoeve A L J, de Haes J C J M 1993 Fatigue in cancer patients. British Journal of Cancer 68: 220–224

Steptoe A 1991 The links between stress and illness. Journal of Psychosomatic Research 35(6): 633–644

Sykes B J 1976 The concise Oxford dictionary of current english. Book Club Associates, London

Theorell T 1974 Life events before and after the onset of a premature myocardial infarction. In: Dohrenwend B P, Dohrenwend B S (eds) Stressful life events – their nature and effects. Wiley, New York, p 101–117

Van Hilten J J, Weggeman M, van der Velde E A, Kerkhof G A, van Dijk J G, Roos R A C 1993 Sleep, excessive daytime sleepiness and fatigue in Parkinson's disease. Journal of Neural Transmission 5: 235–244

Vogel W, Raymond S, Lazarus R S 1959 Intrinsic motivation and psychological stress. Journal of Abnormal and Social Psychology 58: 225–233

Wallston K A, Wallston B S 1981 Health locus of scales. In: Lefcourt H M (ed) Research with the locus of control construct, vol I. Assessment methods. Academic Press, New York

Wallston K A, Wallston B S, Devellis R 1978 Development of the multidimensional health locus of control (MHLC) scales. Health Education Monographs 6: 161–170

Wessely S, Hotopf M, Sharpe M 1998 Chronic fatigue and its syndromes. Oxford University Press, Oxford

Winokur G, Holeman E 1963 Chronic anxiety neurosis: clinical and sexual aspects. Acta Psychiatrica Scandanavica 39: 384–412

11

The ageing process and mental health

The Seven Ages of Man

All the world is a stage
And all the men and women merely players;
They have their exits and their entrances;
His acts being seven ages . . .

At first the infant,
Mewling and puking in the nurse's arms; . . .

Last scene of all,
That ends this strange eventful history,
Is second childishness and mere oblivion;
Sans teeth, sans eyes, sans taste, sans everything.

(William Shakespeare *As You Like It* Act 2, Scene 7)

Key Points
▪ All of the changes occurring in the human body eventually result in diminished functional efficiency and impairment
▪ Exposure to ultraviolet light produces pathological changes
▪ There are age-related changes in the brain that include reduced brain weight and enlarged ventricles
▪ There are several theories that attempt to explain the ageing process
▪ Alzheimer-type dementia is characterised by shrinkage of cerebral cortex and axons
▪ Some pharmacological management of dementia involves the use of inhibitors of acetylcholinesterase in brain tissue
▪ There is a low prevalence of major depression and a high prevalence of minor depression among elderly people
▪ Low plasma albumin as an assessment tool can be due to poor nutritional status, acute illness or immobility
▪ The life of an individual is full of drama and many changes affecting the five dimensions of the person

The life continuum from birth to senescence and death (Fig. 11.1) is characterised by growth and development that encompasses the five dimensions of the human being, which includes physical, psychological, social, intellectual and spiritual changes. Life expectancy at birth has increased for both women and men, although more so for women (Wingard & Cohn 1990). Both the life expectancy for both sexes and the

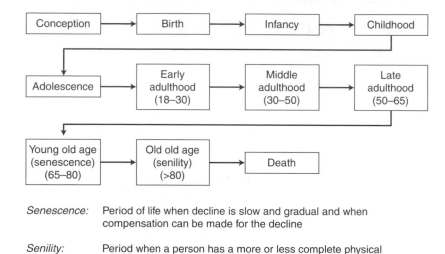

Senescence: Period of life when decline is slow and gradual and when compensation can be made for the decline

Senility: Period when a person has a more or less complete physical breakdown, mental disorganisation and loss of mental faculties

Figure 11.1 The lifespan.

sex differential in longevity must yield enormous personal, economic, social and cultural consequences within the ageing process continuum. While the reader might not agree with Shakespeare's description of the 'last scene of all' in his seven ages of man, there is no doubt that all the changes that occur in the human body with the passage of time eventually lead to diminished functional efficiency and to impairment. Thus, the ageing process in later life is characterised by a progressive decrease in ability of the body's homeostatic mechanisms to respond to stressors (see Chapter 10).

This chapter explores and discusses the physiological and psychological theories of ageing and highlights the characteristics of normal physiological and mental ageing processes. Pathophysiological issues of the ageing process are cited with special reference to brain physiology and pathology. Nursing issues associated with the assessment of functional ability are discussed and aspects of restoration of function/well-being are explored.

CHARACTERISTICS OF PHYSICAL AGEING

During normal ageing, the skin becomes thin, dry and inelastic. Collagen fibres in the dermis become thicker and less elastic. Adipose tissue in the hypodermis diminishes from the age of 45 years onwards and wrinkling, the permanent infolding of the skin due to loss of elasticity and thinness, becomes more apparent. It is now known that some of these physiological characteristics such as wrinkling, pigment alteration and thinning of the skin are not normal progression of the ageing process but are patho-logical changes that result from exposure to ultraviolet light (Bennett & Ebrahim 1995). The dryness of the skin is due to decreased secretion of sebum by the sebaceous glands but, in addition, both the hair follicles and the sweat glands decrease in number. This change in the integrity of the skin means that elderly people do not perspire easily and are more subject to heat exhaustion. The diminished adipose tissue means that there is loss of insulating properties and, coupled with diminished circu-lation, it means that elderly people are also more sensitive to cold. Elderly people also experience decreased metabolism. Grey hair, which occurs in both sexes to a greater or lesser degree, is genetically deter-mined (Bennett & Ebrahim 1995). (See Table 11.1.)

Table 11.1 Physiological functional changes seen with the ageing process. Adapted from Shock (1976).

Characteristic	Approximate percentage of function/tissue remaining	
	30-year-old man	75-year-old man
Nerve conduction velocity	100	90
Basal metabolic rate	100	84
Body water content	100	82
Cardiac output	100	70
Number of kidney glomeruli	100	56
Brain weight	100	56
Hand grip strength	100	55
Number of taste buds	100	36
Speed of blood acidity return to equilibrium	100	17

CHARACTERISTICS OF MENTAL AGEING

The age-related changes in the brain may include reduced weight and volume of the brain, enlarged sulci, enlarged ventricles, and thickening and stiffening of blood vessels and meninges. There are also fewer neu-rones in certain parts of the brain resulting in reduced amounts of neuro-transmitters. Healthy old people experience some decline in short-term memory while long-term memory is not affected, and they also show a lengthening of reaction time, usually by 20% between the ages of 20 and 60 years. However, old people are able to learn, especially when well motivated, and will retain any creative and artistic ability they possess, with later work often glowing with experience. Old people also retain their judgement skills, mostly due to reflection on past experience which often brings wisdom (Roberts 1989).

PHYSIOLOGICAL THEORIES OF AGEING

An illustration of the physiological theories of ageing is given in Figure 11.2.

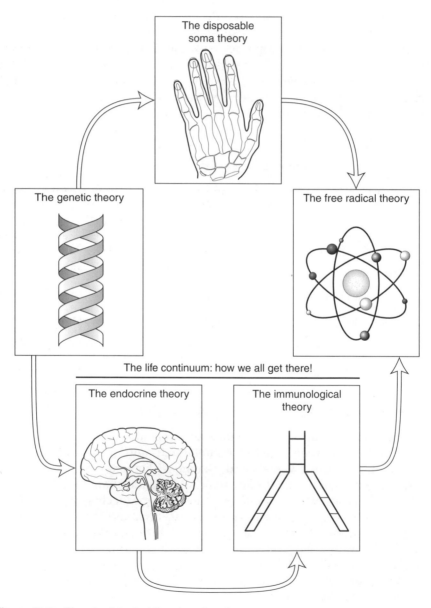

Figure 11.2   The physiological theories of ageing.

The free radical theory

The free radical theory was first proposed by Harman (1968) and is supported by others (Kenney 1989, Kyriazis 1994). The theory proposes that ageing is due to the byproducts of cellular metabolic processes known as free radicals. Free radicals are chemical intermediate molecules containing an unpaired electron which makes them highly reactive molecules. They react violently with proteins, DNA and enzymes, causing significant damage and have been referred to colloquially as 'molecular sharks' (Kyriazis 1994). Environmental issues such as pollution and lifestyle behaviours that include smoking increase the production of free radicals.

Associated with the free radical theory are the qualitative and quantitative modifications of various proteins that occur in various tissues due to oxidative processes and changes in all tissues, but more so in the brain (Beaufrere & Beaufrere 1998). The same authors state that within muscle tissue, mitochondrial and myofibrillar proteins are affected, with the result that there is a loss of both strength and endurance.

The body has developed a system of chemicals known as antioxidants that neutralise and mop-up free radicals. According to Kenney (1989), the role of antioxidants results in the retardation of cellular ageing via nutritional, inhibitional and immunological processes.

The disposable soma theory

The disposable soma theory proposes that it is more economic to invest energy in producing viable offspring than in repairing damaged cells and tissues. For this reason the body is there to protect DNA and is kept in good repair until the time of reproduction when energy use is transferred from damaged tissue repair to the nurturing of immature offspring (Kyriazis 1994). Bennett & Ebrahim (1995) propose that longevity is determined to some extent by the efficiency of DNA repair as shown by the fact that species that are long-lived, such as humans and elephants, tend to have better DNA repair efficiency than short-lived species. The same authors describe the *Hayflick limit*, which is the number of cell divisions that cultured connective tissue cells such as human fibroblasts can undergo before they stop. Moody (1998) reports that Hayflick (1965) noticed that cells removed from foetal tissue will replicate themselves about 100 times before they stop, while those taken from a 70-year-old individual will only replicate 20–30 times. Thus while fibroblasts stop after so many mitotic cell divisions, human cancer cells are immortal since they continue to replicate unchecked.

The genetic theory

The genetic theory argues that ageing has its basis in pleitropic genes (double-edged sword genes) which promote survival in the early stages of life but promote ageing and death in later life. The genetic theory could also be referred to as the evolutionary theory of ageing which proposes that organisms are pre-programmed to age and to self-destruct at some point in time. Other workers (Medvedvev 1972, Orgel 1973) have described what they refer to as the error accumulation theory (also known as the error catastrophe theory) which proposes that random changes that degrade the genetic code additively bring about senescence and ageing as a result of dysfunction in enzyme production. Thus living organisms possess genes that stimulate production of molecules which eventually cause the ageing process. Some food for thought is provided by the accelerated ageing syndromes such as Down's syndrome and progeria. According to Bennett & Ebrahim (1995) the fibroblast cells of individuals affected with these accelerated ageing syndromes show a reduced ability to replicate.

The endocrine theory

As described by Kyriazis (1994), the endocrine theory supports the soma theory and argues that human beings live just long enough to have children and to ensure that their children survive, after which they die.

Support of the endocrine theory can be demonstrated by the effects of the menopause, a stage at which the protective effects of both oestrogen and progesterone decrease. The use of hormone replacement therapy in the form of low-dose oestrogen given over several years starting in the perimenopausal period will reduce postmenopausal osteoporosis and also decrease the incidence of such conditions as cerebral vascular accidents (strokes) and myocardial infarction, which are more associated with the ageing process.

Associated with growth and development are growth hormone, melatonin, other anterior pituitary gland hormones and thymosine. Growth hormone, which is secreted in pulses, shows range, amplitude and frequency that are healthy in a young person while its secretion is less complex in elderly people. In addition, the physiological effectiveness of thyroid-stimulating hormone (TSH), adrenocorticotrophic hormone (ACTH) and gonadotrophins is reduced with progression in time. Melatonin, which is secreted by the pineal gland, interprets the body's perception of the passage of time – what is normally referred to as the biological clock. The thymus gland, which produces thymosine, reduces in size and function with increasing age. Thymosine facilitates the development and maturation of the immune system.

The immunological theory

As humans age there is progressive failure of the immune system, resulting in reduced ability to fight disease. Immune efficiency is affected by stress (Guidi et al 1998, Kyriazis 1994, Leonard & Miller 1995), malnutrition, external damage and decreased thymosine (Kyriazis 1994). Evidence suggests that an inefficient immune system increases the risk of cancer (Guidi et al 1998), autoimmune diseases (Bennett & Ebrahim 1995, Guidi et al 1998), infections (Bennett & Ebrahim 1995, Guidi et al 1998), mental health conditions such as schizophrenia (Muüller & Ackenheil 1995) and depression (Guidi et al 1998, Leonard & Miller 1995).

THE AGEING PROCESS AND PATHOPHYSIOLOGY OF THE BRAIN

The brain of a young adult weighs about 1.4 kg (approximately 3 lb) (Ganong 1989). It is acknowledged that with age the size of the brain is reduced and that its volume can reduce by as much as 10% of that of a young adult (Bennett & Ebrahim 1995). There is no doubt that neurones are lost at different rates in different parts of the brain, with the cerebral cortex, cerebellum, basal ganglia and the locus coeruleus being mostly affected. Bennett & Ebrahim (1995) suggest losses of 1% per year in the cortex and 40% per year from the locus coeruleus of the cerebellum in those individuals aged 60 and above (Curcio et al 1982, Duara et al 1985, Rebenson-Piano 1989). Other changes that can be seen on examination of the brain are enlargement of the ventricles and deepening of the sulci, and prominence of the gyri. Observation of an atrophied aged brain shows several features of ventricular asymmetry due to accumulation of cerebrospinal fluid, increased dead space in the cranial cavity and change in colour and appearance of the dura mater (Lytle & Alter 1979, Rebenson-Piano 1989). The number of dendrites also decreases with age, which no doubt explains the slowing in response to stimuli due to reduced synaptic transmission.

Various parts of the brain perform very specific functions such as: sensory activity and recognition by the parietal lobe; motor activity, attention, behaviour and emotion by the frontal lobe; memory by the temporal lobe; vision by the occipital lobe; and coordination and balance by the cerebellum. With ageing and pathological changes, some of these functions are affected to a greater or lesser extent.

One function that is characteristically affected is that of acute memory. Acute memory loss (amnesia) becomes more apparent with ageing in some individuals and is usually associated with damage or malfunction of the hippocampus, thalamus and limbic system. According to Bennett & Ebrahim (1995), short-term memory may be stored as an electrical potential difference between neurones for a few minutes and is eventually stored within hours as new proteins are synthesised. The observation that some individuals, even in young adult life, have better memories than others may reflect on this difference to convert the potential difference into newly synthesised proteins. Long-term memory, on the other hand, is supposed to be stored in the changes within dendrites and their interconnections.

CHANGES IN SENSORY FUNCTIONING

Some aspects of sensory functioning in relation to the sleep–wake cycle and level of arousal have been discussed in Chapter 9. It can be difficult to delineate the physiological, age-related changes to the pathological, disease-related changes that occur in elderly people. Some visual acuity is lost with normal ageing and hearing impairment is common in old age (Bennett & Ebrahim 1995).

Detailed descriptions of both the ageing eye and the ageing ear have been given by Bennett & Ebrahim (1995). A brief summary of the important changes that occur in the eye and ear is given in this chapter to serve as a reference point for mental health practitioners, since mental illness in both young and old people is characterised by visual and auditory experiences such as hallucinations.

Bennett & Ebrahim (1995, p 15) describe the eyes as 'the windows to the soul', which is very true when one considers the many images that are formed in the eye and interpreted by the brain. The dichotomy between physiological and pathological changes in the ageing eye can be very difficult since both loss of visual acuity and the formation of cataracts are characteristics of both the ageing process and pathology. A cataract is due to an increase in the layers around the lens, resulting in opacity of the lens. Tripeptide glutathione, which is present in high concentrations in the normal lens, is greatly reduced in cataract sufferers. Individuals suffering from diabetic mellitis are very susceptible to the formation of cataracts and abnormalities of both the metabolism and the lens concentration of sorbitol have been found (Bennett & Ebrahim 1995). Loss of fat in the eyelids can lead to drooping of the upper eyelid, a condition known as potashes, and to curling in of the lower eyelid, which causes irritation of the cornea resulting in watering and redness.

Old age is also characterised by some impairment of hearing with 50% of those above the age of 75 years experiencing some hearing impairment. There is an age-related reduced ability to perceive high tones above frequencies of 2000 Hz such as those produced by consonants (Bennett & Ebrahim 1995). From the age of 40 years onwards, degeneration of the cochlea and its neurones is common, resulting in a sensorineural form of deafness called presbycusis. The cochlea is an organ of hearing situated in the inner ear.

Other changes within the ear associated with advancing age include reduced activity of the ceruminous glands in the outer ear leading to dry wax, changes in the articular cartilage of the three bones of the middle ear, namely the malleus, incus and stapes, and degeneration of the sensitive hair cells of the semicircular canals in the inner ear.

Within the mental health arena, paranoia and suspiciousness can ensue where there are communication problems, especially where hearing impairment exists. In addition, hearing impairment can lead to severe psychosocial problems of withdrawal, isolation and depression in all generations but more so in older people. To aid communication, one needs to reduce background noise, obtain the attention of the individual to be spoken to, sit face to face with the person, raise one's voice without shouting and speak slowly and clearly.

ALZHEIMER-TYPE DEMENTIA (ATD)

First described by Alois Alzheimer in 1906 (cited in Hamdy et al 1998), ATD is a degenerative disorder of the brain whose characteristic presenting features include confusion and loss of memory in the early stages followed by personality disintegration in the later stages. Statistics show that one person in 1000 will develop ATD between the ages of 40 and 65 years, and this increases to one in 50 at age 65–70, one in 20 at age 70–80 and one in five at age 80 and above (Hunt 1996). Other statistics suggest that it affects 11% of the population between 80 and 85 years of age and 24% of those older than 85 years (Selkoe 1992). Genetic linkage studies have shown and suggested that in some early-onset families, ATD can be caused by a defective gene on the proximal long arm of chromosome 21 (Goate et al 1989). Other studies have also suggested a link with chromosome 14 for early or younger onset and chromosome 19 for late onset (Isaacs & Roque 1995, Poirier et al 1993).

This gene involvement in ATD is appropriately summarised by Hamdy et al (1998) who confirmed the earlier work of others that there are several point mutations to the amyloid precursor protein gene located on chromosome 21 in a small number of early-onset autosomal dominant Alzheimer's disease families. The presenilin 1 gene located on chromosome 14 shows several point mutations and shows its effect in the majority of early-onset autosomal dominant Alzheimer's disease families while mutation of the presenilin 2 gene located on chromosome 1 is implicated in a small number of Alzheimer's disease families. The apolipoprotein 4 (APOE4) gene on chromosome 19 accounts for the majority of late-onset Alzheimer's disease families (Hamdy et al 1998).

In ATD there is shrinkage mostly of the grey matter (cerebral cortex) but also of the white matter (axons). The shrinkage can be displayed by brain scanning; it is more easily definable in young sufferers and less so in people over 80 years of age. Currently there is no definite investigation in life for the diagnosis of specific types of dementia except inference from scales such as the Hachinski scale (Hachinski et al 1975) and from very specialised investigations such as magnetic resonance imaging (MRI) and positron emission tomography (PET). However, there is evidence of degeneration of neurones and their nerve endings and connections. Enzymes related to the neurotransmitter acetylcholine are greatly reduced in the brains of individuals suffering from ATD, especially in hippocampus. In particular, the amount of the enzyme cholineacetyltransferase is reduced in both the cortical and subcortical areas (Kopelman 1993). Thus, in addition to other changes, cholinergic pathways in the cerebral cortex and basal forebrain are also affected in individuals with Alzheimer's disease (Katzman & Saitoh 1991), leading to cognitive function deficits in such individuals (Becker 1991).

The pathogenesis and biochemical mechanisms of ATD has been described and reviewed by several authors (Rang et al 1995, Selkoe 1992). Mountjoy (1993) identifies the four main pathological abnormalities in the brains of individuals suffering from ATD as neuronal loss, large numbers of neuritic plaques, neocortical neurofibrillary tangles and deposition of amyloid. Characteristic biochemical mechanisms are associated with the neurodegenerative processes seen in ATD. Under normal physiological function, extracellular cleavage processes amyloid precursor protein to produce another soluble protein which does not cause neuronal damage. In ATD abnormal processing by cleavage leads to the formation of a soluble $A\beta$ fragment that causes neurodegeneration and deposition of amyloid plaques. The neurofibrillary tangles are believed to be due to excessive phosphorylation of microtubules and their aggregation as intracellular helical filaments.

Pharmacological management of dementia

The drugs used in the management of ATD work by attempting to increase the amount of the neurotransmitter acetylcholine in the brain, a process known as cholinergic replacement therapy (Burns 1993). These drugs are known as cholinergic agents and their use takes various approaches. Choline and lethicin (given orally) are precursors of acetylcholine and require intact presynaptic neurones to be effective, while anticholinesterases such as physostigmine (intravenous) and tetrahydroaminoacridine (THA; given orally) inhibit the breakdown of acetylcholine (Burns 1993,

Kopelman 1993). Other drugs such as dimethlaminoethanol or arecoline, a cholinomimetic, act directly on cholinergic receptors.

Physostigmine and THA

Both physostigmine and THA are anticholinesterases and prevent the breakdown of acetylcholine (Johns et al 1983, Kopelman 1993). Studies by Johns et al (1983) have shown that recognition memory rather than recall memory can be improved when intravenous physostigmine or oral THA is given. The same authors state that intact neurones are not necessary for the anticholinesterases to be effective. THA is also longer acting and a dosage of 150–200 mg daily may be given.

Donepezil hydrochloride (Aricept)

Donepezil hydrochloride (Aricept) is a reversible inhibitor of acetyl-cholinesterase and is also used for the symptomatic management of mild to moderate ATD. Donepezil is a piperidine-based derivative that is chemically distinct from the other cholinesterase inhibitors (Cardozo et al 1992, Sugimoto et al 1992). Observations by Yamanishi et al (1990) have shown that donepezil is quite specific in its action with a higher degree of selectivity for acetylcholinesterase in the central nervous system than that in the peripheral nervous system. It inhibits cholinesterase in brain tissue but not in cardiac muscle (heart) or smooth muscle of the small intestines, and has a very small effect on cholinesterase in striated muscle. Studies by Rogers & Friedhoff (1996) have shown that plasma concentrations of donepezil were related directly to red blood cell acetylcholinesterase inhibition and to cognitive functioning. The same authors suggest that this close correlation between red blood cell acetyl-cholinesterase inhibition and clinical response may form a good basis for the development of a marker for the effectiveness of the drug. In studies when donepezil was given at a dosage of 5 mg once daily for 12 weeks, significant clinical improvement was seen (Rogers & Friedhoff 1996). Indications suggest that it may slow the rate of both cognitive and non-cognitive deterioration in some sufferers as measured by the Alzheimer disease assessment scale – cognitive subscale score (ADAS-cog; Rosen et al 1984, the mini-mental state examination score (MMSE; Folstein et al 1975) and the quality of life as assessed by the patient (QoL-P; Blau 1977). It has a number of side-effects which include nausea, vomiting, diarrhoea, gastric upset, constipation, fatigue, insomnia and muscle cramps, but there are no peripheral cholinergic adverse effects or hepatotoxicity.

Rivastigmine (Exelon)

Rivastigmine is one of the newer drugs believed to prolong functional ability in ATD. It is indicated in mild to moderately severe ATD. Exelon is an anticholinesterase which is highly selective for the hippocampus and cortex and shows minimal peripheral activity and side-effects such as neuromuscular effects like leg cramps and bradycardia. Published data by Novartis, the makers of Exelon (Novartis 1998) suggest that patients taking Exelon showed improvement in recognition of family members, in paying attention, in ability to tell the time and in concentration. A maximum dosage of 6–12 mg can be given daily, usually in two equal doses, with food. Side-effects are due to its acetylcholinesterase effect and include nausea, vomiting, dizziness and headache.

Oestrogen

Beckmann (1997) reviews the evidence that supports the beneficial effects of oestrogen therapy in the areas of the brain that are associated with ATD. He argues that oestrogen may slow the progress of the disease through the effect of nerve growth factor on cholinergic nerve cells. This is supported by Hamdy et al (1998) who add that oestrogen may cause less formation of senile plaques as a result of decreased deposits of β-amyloid protein. Oestrogen also increases cerebral blood flow via a relaxing factor from the blood vessel endothelium and minimises the effect of endothelin, a blood vessel constrictor.

Non-steroidal anti-inflammatory drugs (NSAIDS)

Karplus & Saag (1999) have reported that the use of NSAIDs may prevent the decline in cognition that is associated with the ageing process. While the mechanism is still not fully understood, speculative analysis suggests that the anti-inflammatory effect of such drugs possibly results in modification of the pathways that are involved in ATD or to the initiation of a platelet effect that reduces the risk of cerebrovascular accidents (Karplus & Saag 1999).

Tacrine (Cognex)

Tacrine prolongs the action of acetylcholine within the synapse by slowing down the removal of acetylcholine by the enzyme acetylcholinesterase (Hamdy et al 1998). There is improvement in cognitive function. Maximum dosage ranges from 80 mg per day to 160 mg per day, though the initial dosage should be small. Blood tests are also important in order to check liver function. Hamdy et al (1998) state that only a third of all the patients who take tacrine will improve.

Nerve growth factor

Hamdy et al (1998) report that nerve growth factor has been found in the brains of people with Alzheimer's disease, with the exception of the area around the basal nucleus of Meynert. Nerve growth factor is believed to be a neutrotrophic factor that could possibly participate in nerve cell maintenance and repair. Unfortunately, nerve growth factor does not cross the blood–brain barrier and would have to be administered directly into the brain or via a carrier molecule. Other neutrotrophic factors are brain derived neutrotrophic factor (BDNF) and neutrotrophin-3 (NT-3).

OTHER DEMENTIAS

The other non-ATDs include vascular dementias (multi-infarct dementia); Lewy body dementias, frontal lobe dementias, subcortical dementias, focal cortical atrophy syndromes, metabolic-toxic dementias and infections dementias. The key symptoms of all dementias include memory loss, especially for recent events, problems with learning and retaining new information, difficulty with the handling of complex tasks, impairment of reasoning ability, impairment of spatial and visuoperceptual ability, language deficits and changes in behaviour. Both the algorithm for the diagnosis of dementia in primary care practice (Gauthier et al 1997; Fig. 11.3) and the global deterioration scale (Reisberg et al 1982; Table 11.3) are useful assessment tools in dementia.

Vascular dementias or multi-infarct dementia (MID)

MID is a result of repeated occurrence of cerebrovascular accidents (strokes) in the cortical and subcortical regions of the brain. In the majority of cases, the cerebrovascular accidents are too insignificant to cause permanent damage or residual neurological deficits. Figure 11.4 shows the stepwise decline or downward escalator decline in MID as described by Roberts (1989).

Lewy body dementias

Lewy body dementia is dementia with early Parkinson features.

Frontal lobe dementias

The frontal lobe dementias include such conditions as Pick's disease.

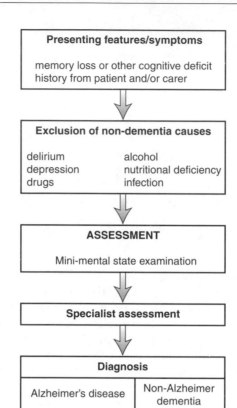

Figure 11.3 An algorithm for the diagnosis of dementia in primary care practice. Adapted from Gauthier et al 1997 by permission of Martin Dunitz Publishers.

Table 11.3 Global deterioration scale

Stage	Clinical characteristics
1	No cognitive decline
2	Subjective forgetfulness but normal examination
3	Difficulty experienced at work, in speech, when in unfamiliar areas, detectable by family; subtle memory deficit on examination
4	Decreased ability to travel, to count, and to remember current events
5	Assistance needed in choosing clothes; disorientation in time and place; decreased recall of the names of grandchildren
6	Supervision needed for eating and toileting, may be incontinent; disorientation in time, place and sometimes in person
7	Severe speech loss; incontinence; motor stiffness

From Reisberg et al, 1982

Subcortical dementias

Subcortical dementias include dementias as a result of Parkinson's disease, Huntington's chorea and progressive supranuclear palsy.

Focal cortical atrophy syndromes

A example of focal cortical atrophy syndrome is primary aphasia.

Metabolic-toxic dementias

Metabolic-toxic dementias are due to such conditions as chronic hypothyroidism or vitamin B12 deficiency.

Infections

Infections such as syphilis, neuroAIDS and chronic meningitis usually do lead to dementia.

DEPRESSION IN ELDERLY PEOPLE

A survey by Ernst (1997) found that while there is a low prevalence of major depression in old age, there is a high prevalence of minor depression and depressive symptoms and a high incidence of late suicide. This vulnerability to depression seems to be related more to physical illness and brain dysfunction than to genetic and personality factors. Ham (1997) has given useful information that can be used in differential diagnosis between depression and dementia (Table 11.4).

Table 11.4 Differential diagnosis between depression and dementia

Feature	Depression	Dementia
Onset	Abrupt	Insidious, no precise date
Duration	Short	Chronic, progressing over years
History	Often previous psychiatric history	No previous psychiatric history
Mood	Diurnal variation	Day-to-day fluctuation
Cognition	Fluctuating cognitive loss	Stable cognitive loss

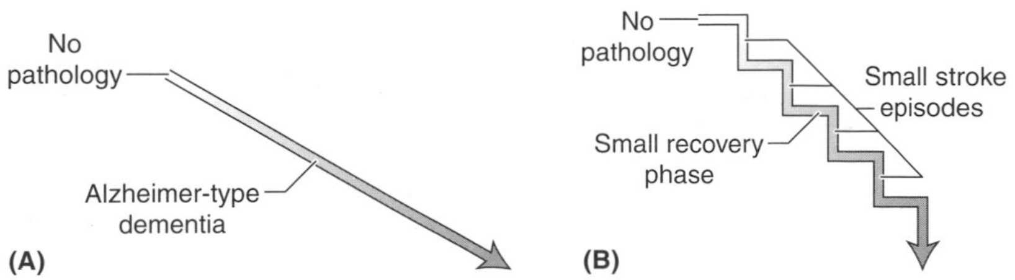

Figure 11.4   The ageing process and pathophysiology. (A) The downward sloping effect of neurodegeneration in Alzheimer-type dementia. (B) The downward escalator effect of multi-infarct dementia (small strokes).

Memory loss	Equal for remote and recent events	Memory loss greater for recent events
Associated symptoms	Depressed mood Anxious mood Sleep disturbance Appetite disturbance Suicidal thoughts	Unsociability Uncooperativeness Hostility Emotional instability Confusion Disorientation Decreased alertness

NUTRITION IN ELDERLY PEOPLE

In 1979 the reported prevalence of clinically obvious nutritional deficiencies in the elderly population in the UK was 7% (Department of Health and Social Security) although this figure could be assumed to be larger now since there has been an increase in the proportion of older people in the population. The issues that need to be discussed here are the frequency of subclinical nutritional deficiencies in elderly people as well as the relationship between these subclinical nutritional deficiencies and mental illness in elderly people. Both these issues have been explored by Morgan & Schorah (1986) who also describe the physical, chemical and radiological indices that could be used for assessing nutritional status in elderly people and the general difficulties in the clinical application of such indices.

Body weight loss, which may be due to inadequate food intake, poor digestion or poor absorption, is the most common index of undernutrition, but it takes time for this to become apparent. Likewise it may take days or weeks for other indices such as folate and vitamin C to be detectable (Morgan & Schorah 1986) and the lack of specificity of such an index as low plasma albumin which may be due to acute illness or immobility does not help. Low plasma albumin due to immobility in long-stay patients occurs because of a redistribution of albumin into the extracellular compartment (Morgan & Schorah 1986).

The importance of mobility cannot be overemphasised, as other studies by Morgan et al (1986) showed small differences in nutritional indices between young people and active elderly people but large differences between various elderly groups. These studies further revealed that the indices indicated a progressive deterioration in nutritional state as the degree of illness and dependency increased. Morgan & Schorah (1986) state that although the mechanisms involved are not clearly understood, some degree of nutritional deficiency is common among mentally ill patients suffering from both acute and enduring mental health problems. While the causal link is difficult to establish, Goodwin et al (1983) reported a relationship between nutritional state and cognitive function in all elderly patients including those who are not ill.

Case study 11.1

James is a 52-year-old grey-haired man who looks distinguished and has worked for many years as a bank manager. He resigned from his job over two years ago as he found that he was unable to cope with his work. Over the past two years he has taken on work at the local post office where he has been sorting letters, but in recent months this has become more difficult for him and he is often misdirecting mail. His wife is in a considerable predicament in that she has been planning to separate and divorce from her husband for some time but now recognises that there is something seriously wrong with him. He appears low in his mood and his wife wishes to be reassured that he is simply depressed because of her discussion with him about divorce. Assessment of his mental state demonstrates that he has some short-term memory impairment, that he is unable to copy the face of a clock correctly, and that he misspells some simple words that, according to both his wife and daughter, he would have had no problem with several years previously. A CT brain scan shows greater cortical atrophy with slightly more prominent cerebral spinal spaces than would normally be present at his age.

He has some depressive symptoms and has been started on Prozac and his mood has lifted although he still becomes very tearful when the possibility of a dementing illness is discussed with him. He clearly is aware of the implications of this and for the moment his wife decided not to leave her husband. He is now off sick from work and seems to be now quite content that his wife is remaining with him, although she is increasingly having to support him because of his deteriorating cognitive functions.

Appetite and food intake in elderly people

Studies have shown that in those individuals who reach old age without physical and mental impairment, there is no change in food intake because most changes in appetite are due to pathological changes that are made worse by other social factors such as isolation, poor housing and poverty (Bennett & Ebrahim 1995). The body's metabolic rate decreases with ageing, especially after the age of 60, but this decline, though continuous, is small. Elderly people living on their own tend to eat simple, carbohydrate-rich meals which more often than not lead to numerous nutritional deficiencies. Physical disability may prevent them from shopping and preparing decent meals. Elderly men who grew up in an era when men did not cook for themselves are likely to have very limited skills and may suffer from 'widower's scurvy' (Bennett & Ebrahim 1995).

Taste and smell perception are reduced with ageing and smoking as shown by the fact that, with the exception of salt taste, sweet, sour and bitter tastes are gradually lost and are important in influencing both appetite and what is actually eaten. In addition, the presentation of the food in terms of its colour, texture, smell, temperature and overall appearance do enhance the wholesomeness of the food and do improve appetite (Bennett & Ebrahim 1995). Poor or absence of good dentition does affect an individual's choice of diet, often resorting to mostly carbohydrate foods or soft foods. Mental states such as confusional states and depression both affect food intake.

The therapeutic value of meals

There is no doubt that in both young and old people, and across the social, cultural, religious, racial and the class divisions, meals are social events. The meal situation in institutional settings is characterised by patients sitting in small groups of four, five or six people. This helps to make eating both more natural and comfortable, even though the patients' eating may be made difficult by either individual handicaps or disease processes or both (Sidenvall et al 1994). This makes the use of ordinary cutlery difficult and reduces patients' eating competence (Siebens et al 1986), as well as the reduced ability to transport food from plate to mouth (Athlin et al 1989), leading to food being spilt onto the table and on patients' clothes (Sidenvall and Ek 1993). The question that arises is how all these problems in eating competence may influence the overall dietary intake of the patient and what can nurses do to improve the situation?

Studies by Sidenvall et al (1994) showed both positive and negative aspects for collective dining room eating. Nurses' interventions by offering feeding cups, special sets of cutlery and a guard on the plate allowed patients to be self-governed and encouraged independent eating, even for those patients who required assistance in cutting up food. The same authors found that some elderly patients were aware of the inappropriate behaviour of others, with the result that their experiences in the dining room depended to a great extent on the behaviour of others. Patients who spit or cough up food or smear it on the table should not be put together with those who are able to eat independently. Sidenvall et al (1994) also state that it is possible that those patients who are mentally aware but lack eating competence may not want to show too much of an appetite and may eat only small portions in order not to expose themselves to too many failures in the presence of others. The nutritional status of such patients does deteriorate (Sidenvall & Ek 1993) and they would benefit by eating in private. Thus how the nurses sit the patients in the dining room is of vital importance for the patients' experience since the sight of inappropriate behaviour causes disgust (Sidenvall et al 1994).

Elimination and the primary causes of constipation

Adequate nutrition of health foods combined with physical activity stimulates motility of the gut. The special relationship between physical activity and gut motility is one of the main factors that influence constipation in elderly people. Bennett & Ebrahim (1995) describe constipation as a word that is used to mean different things, including decreased frequency of bowel actions, difficulty in passage of hard faeces or increased retention of faecal material in the large intestines. The causes of constipation have been well described by many authors and include: inadequate intake of non-starch polysaccharides (fibre) in the diet due to poor dentition; inadequate intake of fluid; lack of exercise; diminished mobility; ignoring the urge to defaecate due to such factors as confusion, immobility, pain or poor toilet facilities; disorders of the gastrointestinal tract such as haemorrhoids; diverticular disease and tumours; metabolic issues; depression; dementia; neurological factors such as spinal cord and cerebral lesions; endocrine conditions such as hypothyroidism; diabetes mellitus; and many therapeutic drugs. The drugs whose side-effects include constipation belong to the groups of analgesics, antacids, anticholinergics, antidepressants, antihistamines, calcium-channel blockers, diuretics, H_2 antagonists, iron tablets and neuroleptics of the phenothiazine group.

Faecal incontinence

The establishment of regular and controlled bowel habits in elderly patients reflects successful nursing care (Brocklehurst 1964). There is a close relationship between faecal impaction, faecal incontinence and diarrhoea, with faecal impaction being the commonest cause of both faecal incontinence and diarrhoea in elderly people (Brocklehurst 1964). Therefore, it is prudent to suspect faecal impaction when an elderly person has faecal incontinence. The physiological basis of faecal impaction and the normal progression of events from impaction to faecal incontinence is illustrated in Figure 11.5. It is important to remember that occasionally, faecal impaction causes subacute intestinal obstruction with faeculent vomiting.

Faecal impaction must be relieved by suppositories or enemas and it is important to repeat the relevant intervention until the entire colon is emptied, since a single enema will empty the rectum thus allowing more faeces to descend from the rest of the colon.

Micturition

It is important to understand the normal physiology of micturition and bladder control in order to appreciate the factors that may lead to and the problems that are associated with incontinence. In infancy, micturition (the act of passing urine) occurs automatically. Urine formed by the nephrons, the functional units of the kidneys, is excreted via the ureters and fills up the bladder. The bladder wall has sensory nerve endings that are sensitive to stretch. As the bladder fills up with urine and becomes distended, these nerve endings in the bladder wall are stimulated and they send the impulse to the sacral region of the spinal cord where they cause a reflex

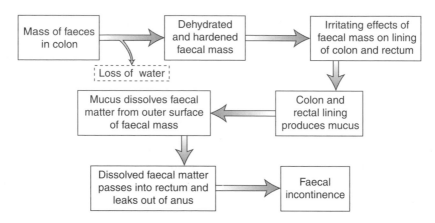

Figure 11.5   The physiological basis of faecal incontinence.

action to occur. Motor nerve fibres from the sacral region are stimulated and they cause contractions of the bladder wall muscle known as the detrusor. Initially the contractions are small but they become stronger and stronger until such a point when the whole bladder contracts and empties its contents. This is the simple bladder or micturition reflex.

With growth and progression to maturity, awareness of bladder sensations is achieved by sensory impulses being transmitted up the ascending pathways of the spinal cord until they reach the frontal cortex of the brain where they are interpreted. The frontal cortex generates impulses that are inhibitory which block the passage of impulses from the sensory to the motor part of the spinal cord. This prevents the build-up of bladder contractions and stops the automatic emptying of the bladder that would have occurred previously in the infant. With growth, emptying of the bladder can be postponed until such a time when it is convenient to do so. With adult maturity the whole process becomes subconscious until pathological conditions alter this scenario.

Problems of micturition

One of the major problems encountered by those who care for elderly mentally ill people, either in institutional settings or at home, is that of urinary incontinence. Quite simply, urinary incontinence is due to a loss of bladder control due to pathological processes and accidents affecting the brain and spinal cord as well as other impairments of the genitourinary system which may create predisposing factors to incontinence. Damage to the spinal cord due to motoring accidents can interfere with sensory and motor fibre impulses leading to loss of bladder control and incontinence. Likewise, pathological conditions such as cerebral vascular accidents, multiple sclerosis and dementia may also lead to loss of bladder control and incontinence.

Incontinence in elderly people can be acute due to changes in environment or to infection of the bladder. Bladder infections cause irritation to the sensory nerve endings in the bladder lining which results in a higher number of bladder contractions that may lead to incontinence. Impaction of faeces in the sigmoid colon and rectum can be a secondary cause of incontinence as it can lead to retention of urine in the bladder with overflow incontinence.

The other factors that lead to urinary incontinence have been discussed by Bennett & Ebrahim (1995) and include loss of mobility, location of toilets that may be too far away, inaccessibility due to heavy doors, inaccessibility to wheelchairs and walking frames, toilet seats that are too low, and chairs that are either too high or too low making it difficult for elderly patients to get in and out of the chair on their own.

Management of incontinence

Acute incontinence is usually managed by dealing with the underlying cause such as treatment of the urinary tract infection. The development of a urinary tract infection can lead to signs of confusion and disorientation in older people with a coexisting organic brain disorder. Other issues relating to management of incontinence and promotion of continence have been addressed by Nazarko (1993).

SLEEP DISORDERS AND AGEING

Some of the issues relating to sleep pattern and older people have been highlighted in Chapter 9. A review of this subject in the literature by Vitiello (1996) suggests that when considering issues of sleep disorders and ageing, the three main areas encompassing all the issues are:

- recognising the multifactorial nature of sleep disorders in elderly people
- the need to treat primary illness rather than secondary sleep disturbance presenting symptoms
- the need to use prescribed hypnotics minimally.

CONCLUSION

Indeed as Shakespeare shared his thoughts in *As You Like It*, the life of any individual is a strange eventful history full of drama and changes that affect all the five dimensions of the person. There is no doubt that with advance in time most individuals will experience diminished physiological and mental functional efficiency while others will show impairment. It would appear that what individuals inherit from their parents combined with their lifestyles will affect the ageing process.

From a nursing perspective, while planning care and deciding on appropriate interventions, it is imperative to think about the possible contributory factors to the specific changes that are noticed in any patient. These contributory factors may have a genetic, immunological, endocrine, nutritional and environmental basis. Whatever the basis of the contributory factors to the ageing process and to dementia, this chapter has highlighted the issues associated with the functional role of neuro-transmitters in dementia and the behavioural changes that are character-istic of the normal ageing process and in dementia. Within the context of this chapter, behaviour is as defined by Hope & Patel (1993), who refer to 'observable acts which can be measured and include activity distur-bances such as wandering, aggressive behaviour such as verbal abuse, eating, sleep pattern and sexual behaviour'.

Knowledge of the pathological processes involved in the different dementias helps the reader to understand the similarities and/or differ-ences in the behavioural manifestations of the various dementias and conditions experienced by older adults. This understanding results in the formulation of appropriate nursing interventions that take into account biological as well as other changes. It does appear that ATD is more com-mon in women than in men, while MID is more common in men than in women (Brayne & Ames 1988). There is no doubt that dementia is more likely to occur with increasing age, whatever the cause may be.

While more focus in this chapter has been given to dementia, it must be emphasised that there are many functional disorders that are seen in old age such as depression, mania, schizophrenia, alcoholism and other conditions. Some individuals may have suffered from a particular condi-tion from early adult life, thus producing a complex picture. For exam-ple, most cases of schizophrenia will have started in early adulthood and, as Brayne & Ames (1988) state, depression is the commonest functional mental disorder in old age.

Most age-dependent changes within the brain are found in the cerebral cortex due to loss of neurones and this explains why higher cognitive functions are affected. Indeed postmortem results show that total brain weight reduces by 5–10% from maturity to about 90 years of age and is most pronounced in men (Perry & Perry 1982, Procter 1988). Thus when considering appropriate interventions, nurses and other health care workers need to take into account all the possible biological factors that may be involved. These factors include the structural and functional changes in the brain itself such as atrophy and other histological changes as well as structural and functional changes in other body organs but with a direct and indirect effect on the function of the brain. The latter include such aspects as deterioration in efficiency of functioning of sense organs, cardiovascular changes, endocrine changes, infective consequences, immunological changes, metabolic changes, nutritional aspects, toxic issues and traumatic influences.

REFERENCES

Athlin E, Norberg A, Axelsson K, Moller A, Nordstrom G 1989 Aberrant eating behaviour in elderly Parkinsonian patients with and without dementia: analysis of video-recorded meals. Research in Nursing and Health 12: 41–51
Beaufrere B, Beaufrere Y 1998 Aging and protein metabolism. Current Opinion in Clinical Nutrition and Metabolic Care 1: 85–89
Becker R E 1991Therapy of the cognitive deficit in Alzheimer's disease: the cholinergic system. In: Becker R, Giacobini E (eds) Cholinergic basis for Alzheimer therapy. Birkhauser, Boston, p 1–30
Beckmann C R B 1997 Alzheimer's disease: an oestrogen link. Current Opinion in Obstetrics and Gynaecology 9: 295–299
Bennett G C J, Ebrahim S 1995 The essentials of health care in old age, 2nd edn. Edward Arnold, London
Blau T H 1977 Quality of life, social indicators and criteria of change. Professional Psychology 8: 464–473
Brayne C, Ames D 1988 The epidemiology of mental disorders in old age. In: Gearing B, Johnson M, Heller T (eds) Mental health problems in old age. Wiley, Chichester, p 10–26
Brocklehurst J C 1964 Treatment of constipation and faecal incontinence in old people. Practitioner 193: 779–782
Burns A 1993 Ageing and dementia: a methodological approach. Edward Arnold, London
Cardozo M G, Iimura Y, Sugimoto H, Yamanishi Y, Hopfinger A J 1992 QSAR analysis of the substituted indanone and benzylpiperidine rings of a series of indanone-benzylpiperidine inhibitors of acetylcholinesterase. Journal of Medicinal Chemistry 35: 590–601
Curcio C A, Buell S J, Coleman P D 1982 Morphology of the aging central nervous system: Not all downhill, In Mortimer J A, Pirozzolo F J, Maletta G J (eds) The aging motor system: advances in neurogerontology, vol. 3. Praeger, New York, p 7–35
Department of Health and Social Security 1979 Nutrition and health in old age. Report on health and social subjects no. 16. London: HMSO.
Duara R, London E D, Rapoport S I 1985 Changes in structure and energy metabolism of the aging brain. In: Finch C E, Schneider E L (eds) Handbook of the biology of aging, 2nd edn. Van Nostrand Reinhold, New York, p 595–616
Ernst C 1997 Epidemiology of depression in late life. Current Opinion in Psychiatry 10: 107–112
Folstein M F, Folstein S E, McHugh P R 1975 A practical method for grading the cognitive state of subjects for the clinician. Journal of Psychiatric Research 12: 189–198
Ganong W F 1989 Review of medical physiology, 14th edn. Prentice Hall, London
Gauthier S, Burns A, Pettit W 1997 Alzheimer's disease in primary care. Martin Dunitz, London
Goate A M, Haynes A R, Owen M J, Farrall M, James L A, Lai L Y, Mulla M J, Roques P, Rossor M N, Williamson R 1989 Predisposing locus for Alzheimer's disease on chromosome 21. Lancet 1(8634): 352–355
Goodwin J S, Goodwin J M, Garry P J 1983 Association between nutritional status and cognitive functioning in healthy elderly population. Journal of the American Medical Association 249: 2917–2922
Guidi L, Tricerri A, Frasca D, Vangeli M, Errani A R, Bartoloni C 1998 Psychoneuroimmunology and aging. Gerontology 44(5): 247–261
Hachinski V C 1974 Multi-infarct dementia: a cause of mental deterioration in the elderly, Lancet 2(7874): 207–210

Hachinski V C, Iliff L D, Zilhka E, Du Boulay G H, McAllister V L, Marshall J,
  Russell R W, Symon L 1975 Cerebral blood flow in dementia. Archives of Neurology
  32(9): 632–637
Ham R J 1997 Confusion, dementia and delirium. In: Ham R J, Sloane P D (eds) Primary
  care geriatrics, a case based approach, 3rd edn. Mosby, St Louis, p 217–259
Hamdy R C, Turnbull J M, Edwards J, Lancaster M M 1998 Alzheimer's disease: a
  handbook for caregivers, 3rd edn. Mosby, St Louis
Harman D 1968 Free radical theory of ageing: effect of free radical inhibitors on the
  mortality rate of LAF mice. Journal of Gerontology 23(4): 476–482
Hayflick L 1965 The limited in vitro lifetime human diploid cell strains. Experimental Cell
  Research 37(3): 614–636
Hope T, Patel V 1993 Assessment of behavioural phenomena in dementia. In: Burns A
  (ed) Ageing and dementia: a methodological approach. Edward Arnold, London,
  p 221–236
Hunt L 1996 Unravelling the tangles of dementia. Independent on Sunday, 28 April, p 42
Isaacs R, Roques P 1995 Genetic link to Alzheimer's. Nursing Times 91(17): 61–63
Johns C A, Greenwald B S, Mohs R C, Davis K L 1983 The cholinergic treatment strategy in
  ageing and senile dementia. Psychopharmacology Bulletin 19: 185–197
Karplus T M, Saag K G 1999 Nonsteroidal anti-inflammatory drugs and cognitive function:
  do they have a beneficial or deleterious effect? Drug Therapy 19: 427–433
Katzman R, Saitoh T 1991 Advances in Alzheimer's disease. FASEB Journal 5: 278–286
Kenney R A 1989 Physiology of aging – a synopsis. Year Book, Chicago
Kopelman M D 1993 The effect of drugs on memory. In: Burns A (ed) Ageing and
  dementia: a methodological approach. Edward Arnold, London, p 193–220
Kyriazis M 1994 Age and reason: theory of ageing, ageing mechanisms. Nursing Times
  90(18): 59–63
Leonard B E, Miller K 1995 Stress, the immune system and psychiatry. Wiley, Chichester
Lytle I D, Alter A 1979 Diet, central nervous system and aging. Federation Proceedings 38:
  2017–2022
Medvedvev Z A 1972 Repetition of molecular genetic information as a possible factor in
  evolutionary change of life-span. Experimental Gerontology 7: 227–234
Moody H R 1998 Aging – concepts and controversies, 2nd edn. Pine Forge Press, London
Morgan D B, Schorah C J 1986 Nutrition and the mental state of the elderly. In: Bebbington
  P E, Jacoby R (eds) Psychiatric disorders in the elderly. Mental Health Foundation,
  London, p 75–89
Morgan D B, Newton H M V, Schorah C J, Jewitt M A, Hancock M R, Hullin R P 1986
  Abnormal indices of nutrition in the elderly: a study of different clinical groups. Age
  and Ageing 15: 65–76
Mountjoy C Q 1993 Ageing and dementia: a nosological and neuropathological overview.
  In: Burns A (ed) Ageing and dementia, a methodological approach. Edward Arnold,
  London, p 1–9
Muüller N, Ackenheil M 1995 The immune system and schizophrenia. In: Leonard B E,
  Miller K (eds) Stress, the immune system and psychiatry. Wiley, Chichester, p 137–164
Nazarko L 1993 Incontinence through incompetence. Nursing Standard 7(32): 52–53
Novartis 1998 Life beyond Alzheimer's – beyond cognition: prolonging functional ability.
  Novartis Pharmaceuticals, Camberley, Surrey.
Orgel L E 1973 Ageing of clones of mammalian cells. Nature 243: 441–445
Perry R, Perry E 1982 The aging brain and its pathology. In: Levy R, Post F (eds) The
  psychiatry of late life, Blackwell, Oxford, p 9–67
Poirier J, Davignon J, Bouthillier D, Kogan S, Bertrand P, Gauthier S 1993 Apolipoprotein E
  polymorphism and Alzheimer's disease. Lancet 342(8873): 697–699
Procter A 1988 Biological factors in the etiology of mental disorders of old age. In: Gearing
  B, Johnson M, Heller T (eds) Mental health problems in old age. Wiley, Chichester,
  p 104–113
Rang H P, Dale M M, Ritter J M 1995 Pharmacology, 3rd edn. Churchill Livingstone,
  Edinburgh
Rebenson-Piano M 1989 The physiologic changes that occur with aging. Critical Care
  Nursing Quarterly 12(1): 1–14

Reisberg B, Ferris S H, De Leon M J, Crook T 1982 The global deterioration scale for assessment of primary degenerative dementia. American Journal of Psychiatry 139: 1136–1139

Roberts A 1989 Mental health and illness in old age. Systems of life no. 178: Senior systems – 43. Nursing Times 85(49): 57–60

Rogers L R, Friedhoff L T 1996 The efficacy and safety of donepezil in patients with Alzheimer's disease. Dementia 7: 293–303

Rosen W G, Mohs R C, Davis K L 1984 A new rating scale for Alzheimer's disease. American Journal of Psychiatry 141: 1356–1364

Selkoe D J 1992 Aging brain, aging mind. Scientific American 267: 97–103

Shock N 1976 The physiology of ageing. In: Vander A (ed) The environment and health and disease; readings from Scientific American. Freeman, Oxford

Sidenvall B, Ek A C 1993 Long-term care patients and their dietary intake related to eating ability and nutritional needs: nursing staff interventions. Journal of Advanced Nursing 18: 565–573

Sidenvall B, Fjellstrom C, Ek A C 1994 The meal situation in geriatric care – intentions and experiences. Journal of Advanced Nursing 20: 613–621

Siebens H, Trupe E, Siebens A, Cook F, Anshen S, Hanauer R, Oster G 1986 Correlates and consequences of eating dependence in institutionalized elderly. Journal of the American Geriatrics Society 34: 192–198

Sugimoto H, Iimura Y, Yamanishi Y, Yamatsu K 1992 Synthesis and anticholinesterase activity of 1-benzyl-4-[5,6-dimethyoxy-1-indanon-2-yl) methyl] piperidine hydrochloride (E2020) and related compounds. Bioorganic and Medicinal Chemistry Letters 2: 871–876

Vitiello M V 1996 Sleep disorders and ageing. Current Opinion in Psychiatry 9: 284–289

Wingard D L, Cohn B A 1990 Variation in disease-specific sex morbidity and mortality ratios in the United States. In: Ory M G, Warner H R (eds) Gender, health and longevity: multidisciplinary perspectives. Springer, New York, p 25–37

Yamanishi Y, Ogura H, Kosasa T, Araki S, Sawa Y, Yamatsu K 1990 Inhibitory action of E2020, a novel acetylcholinesterase inhibitor, on cholinesterase: comparison with other inhibitors. In: Nagatsu T, Fisher A, Yoshida M (eds) Basic, clinical and therapeutic aspects of Alzheimer's and Parkinson's diseases, vol 2. Plenum Press, New York, p 409–413

12

Conclusion

As stated in Chapter 1, the intention behind this book was to provide an overview of selected neurobiological aspects that are important in the overall knowledge base that underpins mental health nursing. In order to assess patients, select appropriate interventions and evaluate those strategies accurately, mental health nurses need to understand the biological basis of mental health problems. As stated Chapters 1 and 2, such an understanding is not synonymous with accepting the biomedical model of mental health. No apology is given for concentrating on biological aspects, for in order to adopt a holistic approach, biological issues need to be considered, reviewed and discussed within mental health nursing. Towards this end, within this book specific aspects of brain function and mental health problems that have particular relevance for mental health nursing have been considered. This chapter serves as a summary of the major themes discussed in the preceding chapters.

The concept of homeostasis, while perhaps more easily understood with regard to physiological imbalance, has been applied to mental health imbalance. Restoration is a key aspect of homeostasis and it is also a key aspect of assisting individuals with mental health problems: assisting in strategies that will help restore rational thought, appropriate perception, the ability to make appropriate choices, a sense of hope and purpose, the ability to enter into meaningful relationships and a positive view of self and the future. Interventions, whether pharmacological, cognitive, psychoanalytical or behavioural, can help to restore mental health either by correcting the altered brain function, by restoring normal neurotransmitter/receptor activity or by developing strategies to deal with altered cognition arising from possible altered brain function.

As well as needing a comprehensive understanding of psychological theories and approaches to mental health, mental health nurses need to have a comprehensive understanding of the structure and function of the brain. A broad overview has been provided with emphasis given to specific regions of the brain, especially the limbic system and prefrontal cortex and to brain neurochemistry. Despite the limitations of the classical neurochemical theories of schizophrenia, mania and depression, alteration in brain function and synaptic transmission are fundamental features of some mental health problems.

Functional imaging data suggest that the pathophysiology of schizophrenia reflects aberrant activity and integration of areas within the prefrontal cortex, hippocampus and dorsal thalamus. Altered dopaminergic and serotonergic transmission has been implicated. There is evidence to support increased dopaminergic activity and sensitivity. Impaired serotonin receptor ($5HT_{2A}$)-mediated activity in the prefrontal cortex has been demonstrated and impaired interaction between serotonin and dopamine has been proposed. However, there is still no clear picture as to the primary neurochemical change that can explain the pathogenesis of schizophrenia.

Over the past decade, attempts to provide a unifying theory of schizophrenia has led to the emergence of a neurodevelopmental origin for schizophrenia. There is now a convincing argument that the altered synaptic transmission and classical brain pathology associated with schizophrenia may arise from some insult during the second trimester or early infancy. This insult may lead to developmental abnormalities which may affect an individual's ability to compensate for and cope with experiences that occur in the context of daily life.

The pathogenesis of depression and mania is also more complex than the simple monoamine hypothesis proposed. Dysfunction of noradrenergic and serotonergic systems is a major feature and, although not fully understood, the interaction between pre- and postsynaptic receptors is of increasing importance. Much is understood about the effects of antidepressants on synaptic receptors, particularly the newer selective serotonin reuptake inhibitors, although the primary mechanism remains unclear.

A broad perspective has been adopted for this book, hence the inclusion of chapters on nutrition, stress, the immune system and the elderly. This broad perspective is also essential for mental health nursing. The physiological effects of eating disorders are well recognised by mental health professionals and it may well be that a specific abnormal gene associated with bulimia and anorexia is located. However, there are broader issues around nutrition that mental health nurses need to grasp. Mood disorders, particularly in children, may arise from food allergies. Deficiencies in nutrients, such as folic acid, may contribute to the development of schizophrenia. Psychological stress may result in changes in eating patterns and mental health nurses should seek to help individuals with mental health problems to achieve a healthy diet. Although not appropriate for discussion in this book, there are moral and ethical issues related to feeding, particularly with individuals with eating disorders and individuals with chronic organic brain disorders.

In keeping with the current demographic picture, mental health nurses will be increasingly involved with assisting older adults with mental health problems. Depression is more common within the older population than is generally appreciated. Mental health nurses need to understand the psychological, social, spiritual and physical issues surrounding the process of becoming an older adult. Specific physiological and sensory changes have been discussed in this book and the pathogenesis of dementia has been examined.

Sleep disorders and the use of hypnotics have been considered in this book. As discussed various factors may result in the transient disturbance of sleep and, in addition, sleep disturbance can be an early indicator of the development of mental health problems or deterioration in mental well-being. Sleep disorders are disabling for carers as well as for the individual. Health care professionals need to be alert to the presence of sleep disorders and to develop expertise in both pharmacological and non-pharmacological strategies to help individuals to resume a pattern of good-quality sleep. Understanding about sleep and sleep disorders needs to have greater prominence in the knowledge base of mental health nurses.

The effects of stress and the immunological basis of mental health problems have been discussed. The influence of 'stress' on the immune system and the role alterations in the immune system have on the development of mental health problems is complex and often confusing. There seems to be a greater understanding of the pathophysiological changes in the brain, initiated by the immune response to infection by HIV-1 and the development of dementia. Chronic fatigue syndrome (CFS) is now recognised in its own right. While its exact mechanism is unclear, CFS exemplifies the interaction between mood, behaviour and the immune system. Again there is evidence to show that there is alteration of the immune system in some patients with major mental health problems such as depression and schizophrenia. Notwithstanding major methodological problems, the area of psychoneuroimmunology could prove to be a fertile ground for research. What does seem clear is that the neuroendocrine and immunological consequences to environmental challenges depends on individuals' capacity to cope with the specific challenge. Mental health nurses have a particular role to help people to develop effective coping strategies that are derived from a rationale that has its basis on an understanding of the holistic functioning of the individual.

Psychopharmacology is an area that in the past has provoked various responses within mental health nursing. A discussion on the current place of psychopharmacology and the use of specific groups of drugs for specific mental health problems is presented. The discussion can never be complete with new drugs emerging at a remarkable rate. What is clear is that the understanding of the biological basis of mental health is in part directed by developments in understanding of the mechanisms of action of particularly newer generations of drugs. Undoubtedly for some individuals, drugs can have a major beneficial impact on their lives and mental health nurses will be involved in the administration of drugs and in the provision of education about the drugs administered. Psychopharmacology is a growing area of knowledge and mental health nurses need to be active in keeping up to date with developments, particularly with regard to the monitoring of side-effects and developing appropriate education strategies to empower clients and enhance compliance. To function as effective advocates, mental health nurses need to have appropriate, evidence-based knowledge.

This book has been an attempt to raise the importance of a biological understanding of mental health problems within the context of mental health nursing. The success or lack of success in achieving that goal can only rest with the reader and in how any new knowledge is translated into improved practice for the benefit of clients.

Glossary

Adenosine Triphosphate (ATP) The universal energy-carrying molecule manufactured in all living cells to enable the capturing and storage of free energy.

Agranulocytosis A serious blood disorder where there is a major reduction in or an absence of circulating neutrophils.

Akathisia A disorder of movement characterised by restlessness and agitation, such as an inability to sit still.

Ataxia An abnormality of movement characterised by a lack of coordination, jerky movements, staggering and postural imbalance.

Choreiform movement Movement that resembles the characteristic rapid and jerky movement associated with chorea. Involves involuntary, purposeless, rapid motions such as the flexing and extending of the fingers and the raising and lowering of the shoulders.

Confabulation The plausible and detailed fabrication of situations and experiences to fill in gaps in the memory.

Dysarthria This is difficulty with or poor articulated speech.

Gynaecomastia Abnormal enlargement of one or both breasts in men.

Hypnagogic hallucinations Bizzare and vivid visual imagery experienced at the onset of sleep, i.e. during the period between wakefulness and sleep.

Hypoxaemia Low concentration of oxygen in arterial blood.

Leucopenia An abnormal decrease in the number of white blood cells.

Lewy body Named after the German neurologist Frederick H. Lewy. They are concentric spheres found inside vacuoles in the midbrain and brainstem neurones in patients with idiopathic Parkinson's disease, Alzheimer's disease and other neurodegenerative conditions.

Magnetic resonance imaging (MRI) Specialised form of medical imaging that uses radiofrequency radiation as its source of energy.

Opthalmoplegia Paralysis of some or all of the muscles of the eye.

Positron emission tomography (PET) A computerised radiographic technique that employs inhaled or injected radioactive material to examine the metabolic activity of various body structures.

Single photon emission computed tomography (SPECT) A variation of computed tomography scanning for the assessment of receptor or metabolic activity. Instead of using positron-emitting isotopes, single photon emitters are used.

Index

C

Caffeine, 48
Calcium, 44–46, 50, 90, 115, 133
Cancer, 22–23, 173, 175, 189
Cannon, Walter Bradford, 7–8
Cannon–Bard theory, 172
Carbamazepine, 136
Carbohydrate craving
  premenstrual syndrome, 69–70
  seasonal affective disorder, 67
Carbohydrates, dietary, 198–200
Carbon dioxide, 9
Caring process, 21
Cartesian philosophy, 16–17
Cataplexy, 160–161
Cataracts, 23, 190
Catecholamines, 90, 106
Caudate nucleus, 37
Cell death, 9
Cell-mediated immunity, 88
Central nervous system (CNS), 27, 28
  control centre, 12
  HIV infection, 95–97
Cerebellum, 28
  degeneration, 116
  neurone loss, 189
Cerebral cortex, 29–40
  association areas, 34
  hallucinations, 11
  homeostasis, 15–16
  motor function, 32–33
  neurones, 31, 189
  sensory function, 31–32
  sensory memory, 11
  somatosensory cortex, 31–32, 35
Cerebral oedema, 9
Cerebrospinal fluid (CSF), 9
Cerebrovascular accidents (strokes), 188,
  195, 202–203
Cerebrum, 28, 29–40
  grey matter, 29, 34–40, 61
  white matter, 29, 34
Chemoreceptors, 10, 11
Chloral hydrate, 157
Chlordiazepoxide, 142
Chloride, 55
Chlormethiazole, 157
Chlorpromazine, 136, 137, 138, 141
Cholecystokinin (CCK), 111
Choline, 49, 51, 192
Cholineacetyltransferase, 192
Cholinergic receptors, 41–42, 152
Cholinergic replacement therapy, 192
Cholinesterase inhibitors, 193
Choreiform movement, 213
Chromosomes, 73–75, 77
  see also Genetics

Chronic fatigue syndrome
  hypomagnesaemia, 114
  immune system, 93–95, 173–176, 211
  and stress, 173–176
Circadian rhythms, 20, 153
Citalopram, 128
Citric acid cycle (Krebs cycle;
  tricarboxylic acid cycle), 62, 114
Clinical ecology, 116–117
Clomipramine, 127, 133
Clopenthixol, 138
Closed systems, 10
Clotting cascade, 14
Clozapine (Clozaril), 136, 137, 138,
  139–140, 141
Clozaril Patient Monitoring Service, 141
Cocaine, 53
Cognex, 194
Cognitive appraisal, 169–170
Cognitive–behavioural therapy, 160
Collagen, 184
Commissural fibres, 34
Communication problems, 190–191
Complement, 90
Concordance, 74
Confabulation, 213
Confusion
  biological basis, 3
  hypoglycaemia, 64
Constipation, 3, 200–201
Coping
  mechanisms, 172–173, 178
  natural killer cells, 175
  strategies, 20, 211
  style, 95
Corpus callosum, 34
Corpus striatum, 37, 52
Corticosterone, 170
Corticotrophin releasing hormone
  (CRH), 37, 65, 177
Cortisol, 65–66
  depression, 65–66, 90
  sleep cycle, 150
  stress, 170
Cranial nerves, 41
Creatinine, 9
Cultural influences, 2
Curare, 51
Cure–care models, 2
Cushing's syndrome, 63
Custodial care, 4
Cyclic adenosine monophosphate
  (cyclic AMP), 50
Cyclic guanosine monophosphate
  (cyclic GMP), 50
Cysteic acid, 49
Cytokines, 20, 88–89
  HIV infection, 96
  schizophrenia, 92